What Doctors Don't Tell You About Tubal Ligation and Post Tubal Ligation Syndrome (PTLS)

What Doctors Don't Tell You about Tubal Ligation and Post Tubal Ligation Syndrome

Must reading for women
considering a tubal ligation,
for women who had a tubal ligation,
and their loved ones.

Susan Bucher

NOTE TO THE READER: This book is an anthology. The information, ideas, and suggestions contained within are for general educational purposes only. It does not diagnose, prescribe or treat patients in any way. The information contained within is to be used as a means of increasing individual knowledge and awareness of medical issues and health concerns. It is not a substitute for the knowledge, skill, and judgment of trained physicians or other health-care professionals in patient care. It is not intended in any way to replace sound medical consultation, diagnosis and treatment by a licensed physician. The author advocates individuals seek medical consultation before making any decisions involving or affecting their personal health care.

The author strives to heighten awareness and advocacy for women's health issues, concerns and rights. If you have concerns or questions about your or another person's health care, please consult a health care professional for advice and health care management. The author, agents, and publishers will not be held liable or responsible for any loss, injuries, or damages (direct or indirect) that arise from any idea, theory, suggestion, or information contained in this book. The author encourages individuals to investigate all resources available and become educated on all topics and health conditions presented to ensure the most informed position.

The author took great care in researching to provide accurate information to support the ideas and theories contained within, but because these anthologies contain ideologies and hypotheses they may be found to be incorrect, and because medical information is continually changing, some information may be, or may become to be, obsolete.

The author does not endorse, approve, or certify Internet addresses and does not guarantee the accuracy, completeness, efficacy, timeliness, or correct sequencing of information located at such addresses. Use of any information obtained from such addresses is voluntary, and reliance on it should only be undertaken after an independent review of its accuracy, completeness, efficacy, and timeliness. Reference within to any specific commercial product, process, or service by trade name, trademark, service mark, manufacturer, or otherwise does not constitute or imply endorsement, recommendation, or favoring by the author.

As of the publication of this book, the conventional mainstream medical community does not recognize post tubal ligation syndrome (PTLS or PTS) as a real and true condition.

First Edition

Copyright © 2006 Susan J Bucher

www.Tubal.org

All rights are reserved

ISBN 1-4116-7504-5

Published by www.lulu.com

Cover design by Susan Bucher
Cover photograph © Sean Locke/iStockphoto.com

For my daughters,
    Zena and Dana.

May you live in a world where women's rights are honored
    and where women are informed.

For all women who have undergone tubal ligation.

May this abusive cycle of non-consent end
    so that your daughters may live in a world
where women's rights are honored
    and where women are informed.

Index

Foreword	1
Introduction	9
Population Control and Public Policies Today	12
Issues of consent, disclosure, and truth telling	16
Truth Telling, Adverse Effects and Medical Errors	21
Primary Disclosure and Secondary Disclosure	24
Diagnosed "627.2" "Post-Menopausal" Then "POF"	29
Tubal Ligation I.Q. Test	33
Post Tubal Ligation Syndrome (PTS) Symptom List	37
Post Tubal Syndrome Examined	43
How Women are Diagnosed with Post Tubal Syndrome (PTS)	51
Hormone Testing For Post Tubal Ligation Women	69
Do Doctors Steal Eggs?	79
The Magic Cure to Post Tubal Syndrome	85
About the Coalition for Post Tubal Ligation Women	87
Letters and Statements to the CPTwomen	93
Actions to Take	115
State and Local Medical Boards	119
There Should Be a Law; Draft of Proposed Legislation	129
IL NOW - 1999 TUBAL LIGATION RESOLUTION	135
Information for Researchers	136
In Closing	145
Web Resources	147

Heartfelt gratitude goes to Dr. VGH, Dr. PC, Dr. S, Dr. J,
Professor V, and countless others (you know who you are)
for providing me with truthful information,
steering me in the correct directions, and
for your insight, support, guidance, and education.

    Thank you.

DOG MA MA

1. BTL has no side affects
2. Your complications after a BTL are all in your head
3. A hysterectomy will cure you
4. Trust me
5. Reversal will solve your problems

ALL ARE DOG MA MA - Dr. VGH

Foreword by, Dr. Vikki Hufnagel, MD

First of all most physicians will tell you that there is no such thing as post tubal ligation syndrome (PTLS). I read So many self help books written by gynecologist's giving advice to women. None of them wrote about this condition. They had to have seen the same cases I saw. They could not be in practice and never have a woman complain after a bilateral tubal ligation (BTL). This was not possible. Women complain and no one listens. Women are nuts anyway is the problem as we are labeled by society, and worse by other women and ourselves.

I commonly heard complaints of pain, bleeding disorders, depression, hot flashes and the loss of sexual desire after a BTL. The most negative discussion I could find was a handful gynecologists claiming that a few women had minor complications.

The routine complications that are discussed with women before their BTL are infection and the risk of the anesthesia . They are told that there are no side effects of the fallopian tube being closed, that they will not suffer hormonal or physical changes, and that their health will remain the same.

Most women are told that they live in FEAR of pregnancy so their life and sex will be so much better knowing they will not get pregnant. It is as if women are stupid and need an operation to prevent them from getting pregnant.

Statistically, the death rate is about 1 in 150,000. This is a low death rate for a commonly performed operation. Women hearing there are few complications and they will be free from worry about birth control get the feeling they are being given a ticket to have great sex. The sales pitch is good. Better sex...no worries.

Yet, what I found was many women woke up from their laparoscopy with some pain and they did well for a few weeks. Then things began to change. The woman begins to complain of climatic PMS and of menopausal symptoms. Women have depression and mood swings develop and they do not associate this with their BTL. A few more months go by and now the woman is experiencing bleeding disorders, and hot flashes or chills.

Within a year many women have lost all of their sexual and sensual behavior. These women begin to lose connection with life as they knew it. They have memory problems and loss of control of their emotions. They will rage and scream one moment, then in tears the next. Often they will lay in bed at night not being able to sleep and then are too fatigued and exhausted to participate with her family or to function at work.

They go to their physician to complain and are referred for psychotherapy. Over and over again these women are told everything they are experiencing is in their "heads"! As time goes on and the cycle continues the women are labeled as "crazy".

Often they are put on mood elevating drugs and anti depressive medications. Husbands are told their wife is suffering from a serious mental condition. Imagine the negative affects on a marriage or relationship when you have turned into a harpy who hates sex.

Desperate and in bad health, losing their minds these women go from physician to physician begging for help and being told there is nothing wrong. Any time they speak about perhaps something happened during the tubal ligation they are informed that is not possible.

I have written and lectured about BLT and PTLS since the 70's. In 1990 I attended the FIS (Falloppius International Society); III. World Conference: Fallopian Tube in Health and Disease. I lectured about "Pelviscopy and Infertility Surgeries and the Need for Appropriate Full Informed Consent" and presented data. I presented national statistics and the need to change our consent processing for women. The French attending the conference spent several hours with me going over the data and working on new consents for France. The US delegates challenged my position which I supported with data from their own organizations and turned to tables on them. I was giving pure statistical data.

By attacking me I was given the opportunity to exposes the abuses I had found in the US as to the many complications that I had found in women after BTL. The data showed many women had pelvic pain, increased menstrual bleeding, mood disorders, and the symptoms of menopause in young women. I reported on my own clinical studies in performing laparotomy on these women and found increased rates of adenomyosis.

I spent many thousands of dollars of my own money to educate the public and physicians on these issues. I spent many long hours and seemed to get no where. The physicians refused to recognize what was happening to over 10% of the BTL patients. The obgyn medical community is not forth coming in exposing the abuses it has created. I reviewed the medical literature and found that some 80% of women evaluated have a serious complication after the BTL.

Tubal ligation has literally been "sold" in the manner of propaganda to women as being 100% safe process with no complications or side effects. As a medical student I can recall seeing women come back to the clinic complaining that they were having hot flashes. Many of these women where young in their late 20's. Everyone of them was sent under the direction of the chief resident to the Department of Psychiatry. Once under the care of a psychiatrists these women are all treated as being "hysterical" hypochondriac females.

Not once did my attending physician (this is the one that is supposed to be teaching you) ever say, "Why don't we run some lab tests and see what is happening with this patient." I instead learned it was easier to write a prescription for Valium which was the drug of choice back then when treating unhappy females. Today the treatments have shifted to Prozac and Inderol. Inderol is given to treat the hot flashes and heart palpitations which get labeled as anxiety attacks.

As soon as I was able to do what I wanted as a chief resident I began ordering hormonal laboratory studies on these women. I hid my subversive activities by over working so no one realized I was actually ordering hormones on routine everyday clinic patients. If I was in an HMO today this activity would result in me being up against a wall in a firing squad. In the past twenty years, I can not recall ever seeing normal physiological levels of hormones be reported back to me in the past 25 years from a woman complaining of symptoms associated with her tubal ligation. Of course I did have some women who are crazy and complained and had nothing wrong but these were with the normal population rates. What I am saying here is the reality is many women are altered by BTL.

I may not like the crazy behavior of some of these women. I have been yelled at by some of them. I have spent hours trying to help them and often even when I succeeded in helping them never got a thank you. They were so angry over what had happened to them that the rage continued as focused on me the one who helped them in the end.

Many of these women do act hysterical. Many are out of control and go from screaming violent attack rage to tearful crying claiming they just want to die. This has not been a fun group of women to work with. Reality is that even psychotic women have physical illnesses, and I have seen and been taught to wrongly label women as has having mental disorders when they had physical dysfunction's (hormonally based and can be corrected) that actually caused mental and emotional disorders. This has happened over and over again. Because of my experience I always listen to the woman first and accept what she says as truth first. This has allowed me to be a much better healer.

I know that PTS is real and hurts thousands of women and I don't care what other physician's think. Everyone; the gynecologists , the American College of Obstetric and Gynecology, the AMA, and Family Planning clinics everywhere has been covering up that complications do exist with tubal ligations.

Post Tubal Women are isolated and discriminated against. Doctors know when they meet a new post tubal patient that she was not entirely informed. They assume that she still is with out the knowledge and it's an unspoken code to never diagnose her condition as being caused by the tubal ligation. If she asks about the correlation she's told it's not possible.

What ever happened to "putting the patient's best interest first" and "do no harm"? Am I the only one reaching for this goal?

For the record PTS is real.

PTLS = Lack of Hormones

Blood test after blood test I ordered on women having complaints after a tubal ligation came back either low or not detectable levels were so low. I do not believe that today's Physicians are not aware of this situation. They are informed of this condition, but are told that it's hush, hush and not to be discussed. To do so is taboo. They fear repercussions from their peers that will ultimately result in affecting their professional status.

Their way they of dealing with the women who return complaining is by simply going along with the party line and blowing off the woman that complains to them. When a post tubal women finds no answers or gets no help they begin to go from physician to physician in a long odyssey seeking to become whole again. The physicians label these women as hysterical and talk about who's office they are going to next.

I have seen women not tested for their hormones for many, many years, but yet these women are offered hysterectomies, D&C's, and other treatments that may be unnecessary, and harmful to treat her condition.

All of these post tubal women are MENOPAUSAL. They are all suffering the surgical castration of their ovaries caused by the BTL. By doing a simple blood test I can offer to re-establish a woman's normal physiological levels of hormones and help bring her back to normal or at least near normal.

What most often has taken place in these cases is that the surgeon has cut, clamped, or burned the blood vessels traveling to the ovary so that the ovary actually loses its blood supply and dies as a result of the tubal ligation. In these cases the ovary simply stops at different rates in the production of hormones, co-factors and other substances that are necessary for normal female functioning.

In other cases the disruption that takes place during the tubal ligation can stop the ovary from producing functional cysts , it can also create gigantic large cysts, partially produce hormones, not produce a corpus leutum, and disrupt the co factor mechanism between the fallopian tube and ovary. These are just a few things that can take place after a tubal ligation that can negatively affect female physiology and anatomy. This is physical interruption that takes place because of physical damage caused by the BTL. The rates of destruction of hormone function after the BTL vary. The ovary can take many months to shut off after the tubal ligation.

You can find out more about PTLS and talk with other women with these problems by going to: www.tubal.org on the web. I also link to this web and write about BLT and PTLS on my web site www.drhufnagel.com under www.nomorehysterectomies.com and www.nomoremenopause.com. Often reversal of many negative conditions are achieved by using FRS to repair the female organs. I have been able to repair and increase the blood supply to the ovary which has resulted in the stimulation of hormonal production.

I treat all of the PTS women as having a form of surgical castration. So a full hormonal panel is ordered and the subphysiological levels are replaced back to reproductive levels using natural cyclic hormones (NCH).

Case Study - Susan Bucher

Susan was only in her early 30's when her tubes were cut and burned. She began to have some symptoms of menopause several months after her tubal ligation. With in two years she was in full menopause and had hormonal levels of a 70 year old female. I saw her ovaries and saw actually where the blood supply had been destroyed by the tubal ligation procedure. She had no signs of any normal ovarian hormonal functions.

When Susan returned to her original physician he did not order hormone testing for her despite her menopausal complaints such as that her menses had stopped. He told her she was too young to be in menopause when in fact she was surgically menopausal, (castrated) and suffering from "hormone shock".

HORMONE SHOCK

Hormone shock is caused by a sudden change (increase, decrease, or interruption) of hormones. Tubal ligations often cause a sudden decrease and sometime full interruption of hormones. This I have seen and is more significant the younger the woman is. Young women literally go crazy and experience shock as their gonads die. Not only are hot flashes common (as with a natural menopause), but so are "chills" which is a more typical repose humans have to shock.

In reading the medical literature the time factor for complete death of an ovary ranges from 3 to 18 months following a tubal ligation. To have all your hormones disrupted does make you crazy. This is not something you can control.

Husbands notice that their wife is no longer the same women they married and think it's because of them. They don't understand why the sweet, loving, great mom is now angry, foul, uncaring and mentally numb. The lack of hormones creates mood swings, fatigue, and lack of sexual desire and depression. The affected woman becomes out or sorts and crazy because she has been made that way "iatrogenic" which means caused by the physician. It's not her fault.

Susan Bucher had her bilateral tubal ligation because her doctor suggested it to her. He sold her on the idea by telling her she shouldn't be on oral Contraceptives long term. She was told that the long term use of these medications would possibly lead to her developing cancer.

Only after some years of suffering did he finally agreed to treat her. In the end what he offered to her for treatment is what all post tubal women are given as treatment... . He offered her of all things to treat her condition : ORAL CONTRACEPTIVES.

Yes, this is an irony with tubal ligations. Many of the women who undergo bilateral tubal ligation are looking to escape from the use of birth control pills and buy the sales job that tubal ligation is safe and with no side affects. These same women if they are lucky enough to get offered any treatment are treated with birth control pills in order to deal with the hormone imbalance that took place.

The cure is the cause. Or is it the cause is the cure?

The physician hears that she's post tubal and that her periods have stopped or have become irregular. He/she prescribes birth control pills to bring on or "regulate" her menses. So the very thing a woman has tried to escape from becomes her treatment/cure for the complication created by the tubal ligation.

*Inexplicable

Strange...but real. And sad.

History

I met Susan Bucher in the late 90's. She was the only woman in the nation to take action against a doctor for not informing her of the risks of BLT and for causing her surgical menopause. I had lost my medical license in California and was soon to lose my NY license. I had no idea a conspiracy to steal my work, income and patients had been formally taking place.

Susan was a classical PTLS case. She went to a California doctor who was to continue my work with a gynecologist on staff and video communications. This never happened. He was only interested in money and not the care of women. He did not properly operate on Susan and caused her great harm. He communicated with the MD that caused her problem and sold her out destroying her legal case. His family is well connected in Ca politically and nothing has ever happened to him for all of his terrible actions. That is another story.

I found that Susan had full menopause and I made the choice to support her and not lie and cheat as the CA doctor and Hospital threaten me to do at the time. I was threaten by this doctor that he would destroy me for not backing him up. He told me that I should "never communicate with Susan again if I knew what was good for (me)." I had come to see he was a liar and a cheat. He cheated on his wife, and his patients. He had used me to steal from me. He operated on Susan to make money and do nothing for her. He made a false operative report.

I spent 1999 working on a book on BTL and PTLS. I had files and papers. I was ready to publish this book and had worked on a multiple book deal with Time / Warner in 2001 to get out of my hell when the California Medical Board (CMB) raided my home and took everything of value from my home. I suspect Caleb Carr had mentioned me to someone to get Warners' to call me . But I was going to have a life again. Then everything was gone. Years of work gone. I am only now able to even think of how to deal with this situation. Everyone was dealing with 9-11. No one cared that I, a private person, had gun carrying idiots of the CMB broke into my home and destroyed my home and my life. No one would ever believe this story.

I had completed NO MORE TUBAL LIGATIONS which was destroyed by the CMB.

I am now in 2006 just beginning to find time to organize things and speak again . This attack on me took some ten years of my life away in many ways. I have a lot of work to heal myself and catch up on my research. I am happy I was always a few years ahead in my concepts so in that way I have been able to keep dreaming. My studies of theology should now become part of my writing and thoughts.

I and Susan have much to offer on this subject . Stay tuned…

Do not confuse birth control with population control. Birth control is what women and couples practice on their own. Population controls are policies set in place by governments. - sjb

Introduction

By, Susan J Bucher

This book is a collection of articles and information about tubal ligation. It contains information about side effects of tubal ligation known as post tubal ligation syndrome (PTLS or PTS), information about the history and politics eugenics, birth control, tubal ligation, and population control.

While some women reading this book will turn directly to the sections outlining the causes and symptoms of post tubal syndrome and its treatment and cures, it's important for women to understand how we came to this point in history where women and the public are not informed of the possible side effects of tubal ligation. We also must consider what can be done so that history does not repeat itself.

It is my hope that this book will not only help educate women and men about PTLS but to also move people to act to cause change. Providing a copy of this book to your doctor or to your state representative may cause them to change how they inform and treat their female patients or to understand that an informed consent law is urgently needed.

Birth Control and Population Control:

Since the beginning of time women and men have sought effective methods of birth control. Birth control is what women and couples practice on their own such as women taking the pill or men using a condom to control their family size, to plan the timing of a pregnancy, or to avoid pregnancy. Do not confuse birth control with population control. Population controls are policies set in place by governments to control the size or growth of a community. Population control programs and policies that stem directly from eugenics.

An introduction to eugenics and population control:

The full history of eugenics and population control policies past and present would be a whole book in its self. Because the endpoint of eugenics is population control that includes tubal ligation (sterilization), it is important to understand the history of eugenics in order to gain a better understanding of why today we are not informed about the risks of tubal ligation.

Eugenics was born and began about the same time and in parallel to Charles Darwin's theories of evolution and survival of the fittest. Eugenics is a term which was coined condoning a reduction in the general population of those who were considered undesirable and a not an asset to society. Right away one sees the ethical and moral questions to this. How would this be done? Who will have the ultimate say as to who is worthy of procreating and who is not? These questions mattered little to eugenics advocates of that time who saw the control of populations necessary to better our human race to be the ultimate answer to future social problems.

Eugenic advocates sought to implement a plan not to kill but to sterilize undesirable segments of the population and restrict them from further procreating so that over time segments of our population would be reduced or eliminated. Grant provided an outline of this in his book, "The Passing of the Great Race" (1916):

"A rigid system of selection through the elimination of those who are weak or unfit -- in other words social failures -- would allow us to solve the whole question in one hundred years, as well as enable us to get rid of the undesirables who crowd our jails, hospitals, and insane asylums. The individual himself can be nourished, educated and protected by the community during his lifetime, but the state through sterilization must see to it that his line stops with him, or else future generations will be cursed with an ever increasing load of misguided sentimentalism. This is a practical, merciful, and inevitable solution of the whole problem, and can be applied to an ever widening circle of social discards, beginning always with the criminal, the diseased, and the insane, and extending gradually to types which may be called weaklings rather than defectives, and perhaps ultimately to worthless race types."

At the turn of the century the science of eugenics became very popular and the eugenics movement was embraced by rich upper class Americans who feared the cost of a welfare state would tax our society to the point that our whole economic system would implode. Private eugenics societies were formed, governmental eugenics record offices were put in place and advocates lobbied for laws that would give governing bodies at the state level the power to petition and order sterilizations.

Pennsylvania in 1905 was the first state to introduce compulsory sterilization legislation. Indiana became the first state to pass a law permitting involuntary sterilizations on eugenic grounds. By the late 20's, more than 30 states had "involuntary" sterilization laws. The targets of these laws included those who were homeless, orphans, blind, deaf, epileptic, in jail, those who scored poorly on IQ tests, and those who were diagnosed as being "feebleminded."

Not only was eugenics a social movement but it was also a "science" related to "education reform". Books about eugenics for teachers and the public were widely distributed. Eugenics became a common feature in college curricula and nearly 90% of high school biology textbooks used through the 1940s had sections on eugenics. Eugenic advocates also played a role in the creation of the first standardized IQ tests. Schools became both the place where students learned basic eugenic principles and where they were tracked for possible eugenic measures.

State officials consistently led the public to believe that the eugenic program did not force or pressure people to have sterilizations. However, reports show when objections were made to ordered sterilizations the victim or their family's objections were nearly always in vain.

After WWII "sterilization" and the term "eugenics" became unpopular with the America public. Hitler's genocide grew from the eugenics movement that was conceived and growing in the west. No one wanted to talk about sterilization or eugenics because of what Hitler had done.

Eugenics didn't disappear quickly. The word eugenics didn't become a dirty word in America until the late 1960s, early 1970s. Nobody was embarrassed to call themselves a eugenicist in 1955.

The American state run eugenics programs disappeared from public view but did not end with WWII. The state ran eugenics programs went underground and continued to operate. The victims were nearly 100% women who underwent tubal ligation.

Information about these eugenic programs is just now surfacing and being reported upon to the extent that governors of states are offering public apology and creating panels to decide compensation. In November of 2002, it was reported that Governor John Kitzhaber planned to offer in a round about way a public apology to the hundreds of Oregonians who were forcibly sterilized by that state. In 2001 Mark Warner and the Virginia General Assembly apologized for that state's eugenics law and hinted that he may set up a memorial to the first woman sterilized under eugenics.

North Carolina had one of the most aggressive eugenic programs after WWII and is the only state to take measures for amends. A book titled, 'Choice & Coercion' by Johanna Schoen details North Carolina's secretive state-ordered eugenic sterilization program. In 2003, NC Gov. Mike Easley publicly apologized for the state's past sterilization program and State Rep. Larry Womble, filed House Bill 1607 which calls for $69 million in compensation for sterilization victims.

Officially North Carolina reports that the last of their eugenics programs were halted in 1974. Oregon reports that the last of their sterilization programs was discontinued in 1981. In total it is estimated that nearly 70,000 Americans (women) were sterilized by "state order". Knowing that some states have destroyed their records pertaining to their state run eugenics programs, it is believed that the numbers of women who fell victim are much higher.

Population Control and Public Policies Today

In American, the state run eugenics programs really did not end in the late 70's/early 80's but were replaced with the creation of the US NSSM 200 and the NSDM 314 policies to control the world's population.

The NSSM was a study done in 1974 by the National Security Council (NSC) entitled "NSSM 200: Implications of Worldwide Population Growth for U.S. Security and Overseas Interests." It detailed the population growth in less developed countries and found it to be a serious threat to strategic interests of the U.S. and the prime cause of political instability in Third World nations.

In 1976 the "National Security Decision memorandum 314" took proposals from the NSSM 200 and made them an central part of United States foreign policy. Dr. Reimert Ravenholt, the head of USAID's population office, made it clear that the Agency's goal was to sterilize one quarter of all women (world wide) and the World Bank explicitly indicated that population control was more important than reproductive freedom.

Originally the NSSM 200 was classified as a secret document meaning it was never intended to be seen by the public. If the information were to be made public it would seriously jeopardize the program goals. When the memorandum was created it was given a declassification date of 1989 but the NSC could have decided to keep it from public view because declassification dates are not mandatory. One reason why it was allowed to be declassified may be the project goals of sterilizing 1/4 of all women had been accomplished. Still, when documents become declassified they are not sent to the press and the document did not became public until 1990 when it was given to the U.S. National Archives in response to a request from a journalist working for the Information Project for Africa. If it had not been for the request of the journalist, it might still be hidden away.

Population control today involves everyone from bodies of the United Nations to UNICEF. It is the specific mission of the UNFPA as well as The World Bank which demands "co-operation" on family planning from leaders of poor nations around the world as a condition of receiving aid and funds. Family planning programs are funded by taxpayers worldwide and pushed by American and Western European political power.

Since the time that the NSDM 314 was implemented all the succeeding administrations have made U.S. economic aid policies to foreign countries dependent on the acceptance of birth control programs. From these policies we have witnessed strict population control policies put in place and mass sterilization of populations in Brazil, India, China, and other parts of the world.

China's one-child policy that was established in 1979 may be the most well known and the most extreme. The policy uses forced insertion of IUDs, forced sterilization, and forced abortion. Family planning workers monitor the menstrual periods for the women in their assigned workplaces or areas. In some places menstrual periods are publicly charted so that everyone can keep track of everyone else.

The goal of the US government to sterilize 1/4 of all women worldwide also included that of women in the United States. The government knowing that men and women in the US would not tolerate being forcibly sterilized as was and is occurring in China, uses policy to control our population by marketing tubal ligation as being safe and that no one is forced because they sign a consent. Stemming from the early eugenics movement through present day MSN 314 policy, the procedure of not providing full information and true informed consent to women undergoing tubal ligation continues on to this day.

Forced sterilization continues in the U.S. because fraudulent practices are inbred in the medical consent process. Not only is there a history of the eugenic movement, advocates and laws being put in place, there is also a history of the medical community which participated in this movement. The roots of eugenics are firmly planted our obgyn medical community as well as in our society.

The eugenic laws that were created in the 1920's essentially gave physicians and the heads of institutions the authority to sterilize their patients, with or without their consent. Little is talked about those who physically performed the tubal ligations, namely trusted health care providers, more specifically, Ob/Gyns. How much were they paid? Who paid them? What effect did it have on the doctors who performed sterilizations when over the decades studies were done and published showing that tubal ligation could have long lasting negative side effects? The studies surely confirmed what those who were performing the sterilizations already knew, namely tubal ligation did have in many cases adverse outcomes. Did the published studies, their personal observations, or their personal bias and greed have any effect or bearing on their involvement and role in the informed consent process for sterilizations?

When the last of the state eugenics programs ended, did the doctors who routinely performed tubal ligations also end their practice of persuading women to have tubal ligations? The answer is no. The eugenic and misogynist attitudes of the Ob/Gyn medical community who at the turn of the century and through the decades performed these operations have not changed.

While eugenic family planning advocates saw and still see value in the surgery, those that performed the surgery also still see value. While Ob/Gyn doctors may have their own eugenics biases, they also have a personal financial gain in sterilization. As explained more in detail later, doctors profit from the original surgery, as well as surgeries that occur from the adverse side effects.

The American College of Obstetricians and Gynecologists (ACOG) was founded in 1951. At their web site the ACOG states that their work is focused in four areas:

1. Serving as a strong "advocate" for quality health care for women.
2. Maintaining the "highest standards" of clinical practice and continuing education for its members.
3. Promoting "patient education" and stimulating patient understanding of and involvement in medical care.
4. Increasing "awareness" among its members and the public of the changing issues facing women's health care.

I have much appreciation for all doctors and the medical world, but when it comes to the issue of the ACOG, obgyn doctors, and tubal ligation, all appreciation is lost and my trust is destroyed. Doctors who were and are on the front line and promote(d) and perform(ed) tubal ligations did not change what they were doing but continued as normal.

While over the years the pill, IUDs, and other methods of birth control became available, the most popular method of birth control for women over the age of 30 remains to be tubal ligation.

In 2000, the journal Fertility and Sterility it was reported that sterilization has become the number one form of contraception in the United States, surpassing even the Birth Control Pill in popularity. Reasons to what factors led to this dramatic increase were theorized by researchers Dr. Carolyn Westhoff and Dr. Anne Davis of Columbia University in New York in their report to the safety of anesthesia and the surgery and because women worry about the health effects of the birth control pill.

My speculation that tubal ligation is so popular because it is marketed as being the perfect birth control without side effects for women who don't want children, or who are done having children.

Today it's believed that women in the US today give consent when undergoing tubal ligation surgery. Women believe that their decision is made upon their personal birth control needs only and her consent is given upon receiving information presented to her by her physician.

When it is learned that information is withheld about negative physical and hormonal side effects known by the medical community as post tubal syndrome (PTS) it becomes evident and clear that consent is given under false pretenses. Withholding information constitutes forced (fraudulent) consent.

Women in the USA today when learning how they were forcibly sterilized by having information withheld from them do not always equate this to having been a victim of fraud or physical assaulted because they were not carried away forcibly to the operating table. Women in the US are lead to the operating table with a blindfold on.

There is a big difference between consent and informed consent. The later includes giving information. While women in the US and elsewhere may sign a document stating they give consent, this does not guarantee that she has been informed or is giving informed consent.

The issue of withholding information and other abuses surrounding tubal ligation are happening worldwide. One situation is that of Peru. While sterilization has been legal in the US for over 100 years, sterilization only become legalized in Peru in 1995. After it became legal, reports were made of state-sponsored health-care providers coercing women into sterilizations with threats and insults, bribes of money and food and failed to provide accurate information or adequate care. The forced sterilization campaign of Peruvian women was documented and reported upon by the Center for Reproductive Law and Policy, based in New York. As a result, provisions to ensure informed consent were established in 1999. Still, women in Peru today, as well as women in other countries world wide are not informed of the known risks of tubal ligation.

Why is full information not provided? The reason is simple. It is difficult to promote and profit from tubal ligation, (whether from one woman or as a whole society/population) unless the recipients can be persuaded that it is safe and intended for their benefit.

Ethics:
Issues of Consent, Disclosure, and Truth Telling

The "one child" policy of China is one of the most extreme and best known forms of governmental population control today. Today we hear and read reports of how women in China have been (and still are) forcibly sterilized. Imagine the horror, a warrant for not your arrest, but for your sterilization. Being forcibly carried away against your will by government police and forced to undergo surgery.

On March 8, 2005, regarding involuntary sterilization, an unanimous three-judge panel of the 9th Circuit U.S. Court of Appeals stated, "Involuntary sterilization irrevocably strips persons of one of the important liberties we possess as humans: our reproductive freedom".

In the USA, it is thought that women are not involuntarily sterilized but I equate having information withheld from me and being told that tubal ligation would not affect my health to what occurs to a woman in China being forcibly sterilized or to women/girls not being allowed to attend school or be educated.

For women in China who are forced to be sterilized, their assaults are ordered. It occurs in broad daylight. It takes more then one person to carry it out. They know they were assaulted and the victim of battery, there is no question.

For women under other repressive governments, they know that they are not allowed information or an education.

Women in the United states, when learning how they were forcibly sterilized by being coerced and lied to don't equal this to having been assaulted. Because we are an educated nation, women in the US don't understand that they, in this instance, have been denied the right to information, education, and their civil/human rights.

It is worse for US women because they do not understand their health changes, and when they do ask about the tubal creating a change they are again lied to and the cycle continues.

The "How could I have been so Stupid" Syndrome

More then once I have heard women make the comment "I wished I had researched more before I had my tubal ligation" or "how could I have been so stupid?". They infer and feel that it is their fault that they were not informed.

As young girls we are taught to be forgiving and say, "I'm sorry" at a young age. For some reason, it is typical thinking for women that when bad things happen it is because they are somehow or some way at fault. It's the "where did I go wrong" syndrome. Women do not recognize, or it is too painful for them to acknowledge, that the doctor that they trusted with intent misinformed them about adverse side effects to coerce/convince them into having the tubal ligation.

For the average woman, researching for information about adverse side effects to tubal ligation on their own would not have helped them. They would not have found information about adverse outcomes to tubal ligation from any common public source. It is not their fault that they were not informed because all information is withheld on purpose from them and from the public at large.

When I was first putting together www.tubal.org, Dr. Hufnagel told me to search everywhere for information about tubal ligation. What information was presented to the public? What laws are in place regarding tubal ligation and informed consent? I searched public library references, medical web sites, and law books. I even searched medical textbooks. What I found was nothing! There are no laws in place and there is no information presented to the public about post tubal syndrome. The only place I found information about negative side effects were from Dr. Hufnagel and her book "No More Hysterectomies", a medical essay text book I found from an antique store dated 1931 (see photo on page 27), and from documents online provided by Grateful Med (now known as Medline). www.nlm.nih.gov and www.ncbi.nlm.nih.gov

The documents that are currently presented at Medline were not made public until just a few years ago with the passing of the freedom of information act that consumer rights activist, Ralph Nader, fought for. Essentially, what was occurring was the government had been gathering and creating a database of medical information. This database was paid for and supported by the taxpayers, but the information that this database existed and access to the database was not provided to the taxpayers. If the freedom of Information act had not passed the information provided at Medline would still be hidden away.

Today when looking at what's presented at Medline it's noted that many of the documents that pertain to side effects to tubal ligation list only the title of the article but do not include an abstract or summary. This makes gathering information for the average person today still difficult and costly. Women with internet access before Grateful Med or Tubal.org was put in place would not have found information about post tubal syndrome. Women today without access to the Internet are not likely to find any information at all about PTLS.

The ACOG reasons it is O.K. not to inform women of PTS because they point to the studies that conclude that there are no adverse effects. One has to question these studies. Are the studies that claim there are no side effects related to or funded by those who profit from doing tubal ligation? Are these studies trustworthy? Are statistics lied about? Andrew Goliszek in his book, In the Name of Science, shows how and why this is done and how our government has tolerated non-consent in a number of experiments meant to control or reduce the population. The government's tolerance of allowing our US women's health professionals to withhold information and allow non-consent to tubal ligation is not only tolerated but I believe encouraged. The ACOGs action of refusing to acknowledge the studies could be compared to when the tobacco companies stated that smoking had no effects. They knew the studies were there but refused to acknowledge them. The ACOG knows of the studies that show adverse outcomes but refuses to acknowledge them or to provide the information to the public.

Doctors today do not fear reprisal for committing fraud and withholding information because they feel that they are protected. They are protected by knowing the US and other governments likes tubal ligation, and protected because all their peers do the same (namely perform tubal ligation without providing disclosure and proper informed consent). These doctors know that in order to be sued a peer must blow the whistle and testify against them in court. It is hard to find someone to blow the whistle when all those that would be called to testify are doing the same thing. Also when doctors blow the whistle on their peers they are often professionally (and sometime physically) attacked, black listed, and made an example for others to be silent. There are laws in place that are to protect whistle blowers, but just as there are laws and court orders of protection to protect women from abusive husbands/boyfriends the law/orders often don't provide the protection needed.

Dr. Hufnagel, an OBGYN, was made an example for blowing the whistle on her peers. She was the first MD to come forth and fully expose and document the massive female surgical abuses in the United States. She worked with CA Senator Diane Watson (now Congresswoman Watson) to put in place the nation's first informed consent law, Senate Bill 835

(Informed Consent to Hysterectomy). She authored "Hysterectomies in the United States, 1965-1984, Vital & Health Statistics; U.S. Department of Health and Human Services, December 1987" and provided testimony before the U.S. Congress. When the document was originally written it contained information about tubal ligation, post tubal syndrome, and how tubal ligations affected the rate of hysterectomies. The document was edited to not include information about tubal ligation. "I was told this information could not and would not be made public" explains Dr. Hufnagel.

In 1989 she went on to publicly disclose information about negative effects of tubal ligation in her book, "No More Hysterectomies" and in 1990 presented information about post tubal syndrome and the need for Appropriate Full Informed Consent at the FIS (Falloppius International Society); III. World Conference: Fallopian Tube In Health and Disease. At this conference the information she presented was welcomed by the Europeans, while her US peers responded with indignity. By her peers she was exhorted and again warned to stop exposing that tubal ligation had negative side effects.

Books have been written and movies made that detail the abuses that occur to whistle-blowers. Examples include "The Insider" and "Karen Silkwood". Whistle blowers are often harassed, threatened, victimized, and fired from their employment. The abuses that Dr. Hufnagel has faced for blowing the whistle on the American College of Obstetricians and Gynecologists and her Ob/Gyn peers for their routine practice of performing unnecessary hysterectomies and withholding information regarding side effects of tubal ligation have been no different. She continues to suffer the backlash to this day.

In 1998, at the direction and assistance of Dr. Vicki Hufnagel, I created the Coalition for Post Tubal Women (CPTwomen) and put in place the first web site dedicated to fully addressing the issues of post tubal syndrome, the continuing practice of forced sterilization, and the need for proper informed consent. Prior to this there was NO information on the web about negative side effects of tubal ligation.

Today the CPTwomen receives thousands of reports monthly from women who were not informed of the risks of tubal ligation and reports of documents being presented for signature while women are in labor or surgery. One such account is what occurred to Barbara O, of Texas in 2003.

"During my labor I was told I needed an emergency c-section, that we had to hurry and that I would be taken to the surgical room after I signed c-section release paperwork. The pace in the room immediately picked up. I was scared and on medication. The nurse came in and pointed to where I was to sign. I was not given time and was not in my right mind to review the documents that I was signing.

Afterwards I learned that I signed an authorization for tubal ligation. Not only was I not informed about the risks of tubal ligation, I was not informed that I was consenting to or authorizing a tubal ligation".

No one should be fooled by U.S. states declaring that their state run eugenic sterilization programs ended in 1974 or 1981. Forced sterilizations continue to occur in the United States and will continue until proper laws are put in place to protect women at the time of consent.

If tubal ligation were not a surgery involving birth control would the side effects would be disclosed? Yes. Do I think that it is a conspiracy? Yes I do, and I am not the only one. Women having tubal ligations and not being informed of the risks is just one example among many other actions that have been taken by our governing institutions as shown in Andrew Goliszek book, "In the Name of Science".

It would have made no difference if a woman did research on her own. She is not informed because with intent the information is withheld. Doctors profit from the surgery and want women to consent and the government supports the hiding of this information. While it is ethically, morally, and legally wrong, information is withheld from women and the public to make us ignorant so we will willingly consent. It is not the first time in history that an abusive medical practice has been waged upon the public. What is staggering is the numbers of women who have been sterilized and that the abuse of withholding information has continue for so long.

Truth Telling;
Adverse Effects, Outcomes and Medical Errors

For doctors informing patients, the issues of consent, truth telling, and disclosure involve trustworthiness and honesty. These are core interpersonal values that are derived from the ethical and morals of veracity (truth) and include the obligations of "respect owed to others" and "fidelity" (being loyal and faithful). These are all principles that are tied into the "Hippocratic Oath", medical ethics, morals and standards.

Respect for others is from the ethical principle of autonomy (freedom/self-rule). It involves the individual's right to be self-determining and imposes on health care providers the responsibility and obligation to provide sufficient information so that the patient can make informed health decisions. Fidelity means being faithful and devoted. In patient/doctor relationships there is always an understanding or implied contract that both parties are being honest and respect each other. From the patients point of view, veracity includes the assumption that the doctor is devoted to the patients good health and best interests and will not lie, withhold important information, or act unethically for their own gain.

Doctors are obliged to discuss with patients any medical research about the probabilities of harm and benefit that may result from a treatment. (Gillon R: Medical ethics: Four principles plus attention to scope. Br Med J 1994;309(6948):184-88.)

Women, in the process of making a decision about if they wish to have a tubal ligation are ethically and legally entitled to sufficient information to evaluate the therapeutic options, evaluate the risks and side effects, and make choices consistent with their goals and values.

How information regarding side effects to tubal ligation is obtained, protected and shared often creates an ethical dilemma and conflict for health care professionals. Decision-making and informed consent is only possible if information is disclosed.

Doctors on a daily basis internally debate their obligations of disclosure with their personal biases, beliefs, and understanding of beneficence and nonmaleficence. Nonmaleficence means not harming patients unnecessarily when providing care and beneficence involves using safe and effective interventions/treatments to care for patients. The principles of beneficence and nonmaleficence involve providing "net benefit over harm" to patients.

Based on the medical principles of beneficence and nonmaleficence doctors consider it O.K. to minimize risks and at times withhold information from patients. They ask themselves how much information should they disclose to help a patient understand (which leads to self-determination). How much information does the patient want to know? What are the potential harms of anxiety and stress that disclosure may cause? Usually this argument of how much to tell a patient is waged when someone is in a life or death situation and not when the patient is in the situation of deciding to have a tubal ligation.

An example may be such as the following: A young woman is diagnosed with cancer. The doctor knows that the patient has a very good chance of surviving and leading a long life but the treatment (chemo/radiation treatment) will most certainly leave the patient infertile plus an adverse effect may occur (such as extreme swelling of an arm/limb as occurs with mastectomy). The doctor believes that the final outcome or net benefit (a long life) is greater then the harm that could occur with full disclosure. The doctor does not want to harm the patient by causing more stress and anxiety, and does not want the patient to delay or forgo the treatment because he knows the treatment will work. The doctor justifies it as being ethically and morally O.K. to minimize the risks and to withhold information about the harm the procedure or treatment could cause.

The doctor may decide to disclose but minimize the risk of a limb swelling because if that should occur it certainly would need to be addressed. He decides to withhold the information about becoming infertile because he considers the woman becoming infertile not an immediate issue such as a limb swelling. He may feel that in telling her this information it would cause undue stress and anxiety (harm) in what is already a stressful situation for the young woman to begin with. The doctor might also think that the possibility of her ever being diagnosed as being infertile and having it be proven as an adverse outcome to his treatment would be difficult.

Adverse outcomes are unintended negative results of medical care/treatment that potentially or actually harm the patient. An adverse outcome can be the result of carelessness or it may be a foreseen but unavoidable risk even when the standard of care was practiced (such as in the case with tubal ligation). The known side effects (adverse outcomes) of tubal ligation are different from medical errors because medical errors are considered to be avoidable. The damage that occurs with tubal ligation occurs with the standard of care because it is the nature of the surgery (to cut/crimp/remove fallopian tube) that causes the adverse outcome. Risks and possible outcomes that are negative but unavoidable become adverse outcomes.

The courts agree that doctors have an obligation to disclose adverse outcomes and have imposed fiduciary "obligations of disclosure" on physicians. Judicial reasoning is that the obligation exist when "one party is dependent on another for information or knowledge that only the first party possesses." (Vogel and Delgado, 66-67).

Because obgyn doctors have knowledge and information about adverse outcomes to tubal ligation and because they have a history of withholding this information, one has to question what is a doctor's reasoning/justification for doing so.

Is it eugenics and bias thinking on the part of the doctor?

"This person does not deserve to (further) procreate."

Is it greed?

"If I inform her she may not consent to the surgery and I will not profit."

Is it a misogynist view?

"She is a woman and not worthy and undeserving of being informed."

Is it that they are apathetic?

"I don't care about this person."

Do they believe that the benefits (no more children) are more beneficial to the woman than the potential adverse outcomes/harm (hormonal imbalance, sudden menopause, bleeding disorders, disharmony with their personal and work relationships due to negative health changes?

Is it that they were taught or feel pressured into not disclosing this information?

Is it a combination of some or all?

Primary Disclosure and Secondary Disclosure

Disclosure can happen at the time of informed consent (such as at the time of or before a tubal ligation) and can occur after consent such as when a patient suffers an adverse effect. I have coined the terms "primary disclosure" as being the disclosure which occurs before a procedure or treatment and "secondary disclosure" being disclosure that occurs at a later time. Secondary disclosure would be a doctor saying, "You are suffering an adverse outcome which was told to you as being a possible risk". As you can see, without primary disclosure occurring conflict and dilemma occurs for doctors in the position of providing secondary disclosure.

For doctors treating post tubal women the conflict of providing secondary disclosure creates moral and ethical dilemmas because they know that the woman did not have primary disclosure. This makes having to provide secondary disclosure much more difficult. Doctors again ask themselves; how much information should I disclose to help the patient understand? How much information does the patient want to know? What are the potential harms of anxiety and stress that disclosure may cause?

The dilemmas of providing secondary disclosure are so great that doctors often avoid medical testing and providing a diagnosis because they fear being put in the position of having to provide secondary disclosure. They do not want to be asked the question "Could there be a correlation to the tubal ligation and my current health condition", which is an outright request for disclosure.

It must be pointed out who most likely would be in the position of having to provide secondary disclosure to a post tubal women, namely an obgyn doctor.

The obgyn in the position of providing the secondary disclosure may or may not be the doctor who originally performed the tubal ligation. If he isn't the doctor who performed her tubal ligation changes are the doctor (being an obgyn) suggests and performs tubal ligation on a regular basis and is also guilty of not providing primary disclosure. Furthermore, the doctor would not want some other doctor to provide secondary disclosure to one of his past patients. This creates a code of silence.

The CPTwomen receive reports daily of what doctors tell women suffering PTS. Only on very rare occasions do women state that their doctor said their condition could have been caused by her tubal ligation. Most of the time women are told that their health condition(s) are due to stress, age, going off the pill, environmental toxins, anything and everything except in correlation to the tubal ligation.

We have received reports of young women listing their menopausal health symptoms (hot flashes, irregular cycles, night sweats, etc...) to their doctors only to be told, "You are not suffering a hormonal imbalance" and "you are too young to be in menopause". This is told to them without hormone testing and when the woman requests hormone testing they are told no.

In some cases the doctor may not provide secondary disclosure because they fear malpractice litigation (if they were the doctor who performed the tubal ligation and did not inform). Or they may fear backlash from their peers in doing so.

The obligation to disclose information rests on both ethical and legal foundations but ask any woman today what she was told of tubal ligation in advance and you'll learn that adverse outcomes such as ovarian isolation (causing ovarian failure/hormonal imbalance) and bleeding disorders leading to hysterectomy are never disclosed.

The ACOG and doctors today state that women are informed because they sign what is called an "informed consent" document before their tubal ligation. These doctors know that disclosure is a central part of the "informed consent" process and that informed consent is more then just signing a piece of paper.

Informed consent involves two things:
1. Telling the patient what the recommended procedure is (and alternative procedures or treatments) AND
2. Telling the patient the risks (disclosure of actual and possible adverse effects) and the benefits.

In the case of tubal ligation women sign a consent document without disclosure of adverse outcomes. They are told and understand the part of the "procedure" being a tubal ligation, and the benefits, but are not told of the actual and possible risks.

Signing a consent document from the patient's point of view is like signing a document stating that you "trust" the doctor.

The action of signing a consent document it is as the patient is saying:
1. I trust that you are going to perform the procedure you told me of.

2. I trust that you told me everything I need to know including the possible risks.
3. And I agree and consent to this procedure because of #1 and #2 above.

    The connection of signing an informed consent document showing patient trust to the doctor brings us back again to the core interpersonal values that derive from the ethical and moral of veracity (truth) that includes the obligations of "respect owed to others" and "fidelity".

    The action of giving consent is not just trust that the doctor explained the procedure and risks, but trust that the doctor (has and) will exercise all due care in treating the patient and trust that the doctor will, if any of the foreseen but unintended harms should occur will be disclosed so that the patient can mitigate the negative consequences.

    How can a doctor exercise due care and disclose an unintended harm if he did not provide primary disclosure, (or if he knows it was not provided)?

The issue is Information and Informed Consent

    It is believed that women in the US today, when having a tubal ligation, give "consent" to the surgery. When it is learned that information is withheld to women about side effects commonly known by the medical community as "post tubal syndrome" (PTS), it becomes evident and clear that consent is given under false pretenses.

    Women today when learning how they were forcibly sterilized by having information withheld to them do not always equate this to having been assaulted because they were not carried away forcibly to the operating table. Women in the US have been lead, and continue to be lead to the operating table with a blindfold on.

---

* Reference. United States Department of Commerce, Bureau of the Census. Reference Data Book and Guide to Sources, Statistical Abstract of the United States. Washington, DC: United States Government Printing Office. 1990 (110th Edition). Table 99, "Contraceptive Use By Women, 15-44 Years Old, By Age, Race, Marital Status, and Method of Contraception: 1982."

STERILIZATION 751

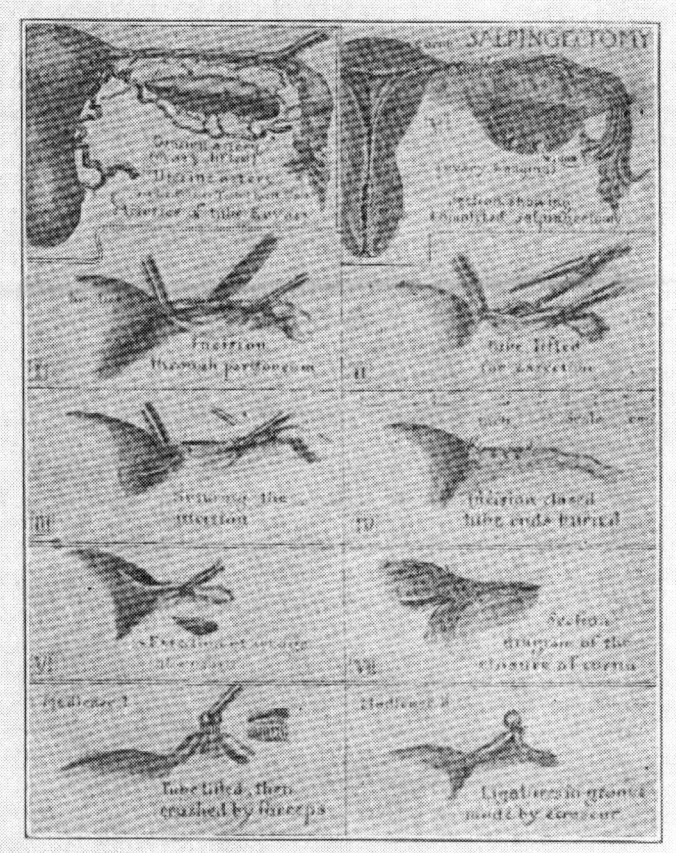

Fig. 165—Methods of salpingectomy: The arterial circulation is shown to demonstrate that total removal of the tube may cause a menopause by cutting off the ovarian blood supply. Even puckering of the broad ligament by mass ligature may do this. As Fredet depicts some main ovarian arteries that are very small, attention is drawn to the danger of ovarian atrophy from checking the chief blood supply if one catches the uterine artery beneath the cornu with ligature or suture when ligating a tube near the cornu or when removing a wedge. Note the marked vascularity of the angle of the uterus, which explains some hemorrhages during or following the wedge operation, especially with excision by the vaginal route. I to V, steps in exsection-ligature. V, diagram showing cut ends buried in the broad ligament under the peritoneum. The spindle canal in the interstitial portion is average anatomy (Guyon's thèse de Paris, 1859). The cervix is from Stieve's Halsteil der Gebaermutter, 1927. VI, VII, the wedge operation, shown in perspective and section. The Madlener écraseur and double ligature is the simplest and speediest of accredited methods. Walthard's larger bite of the tube may jeopardize the ovarian circulation.

"Removal of a wedge at the horn of the uterus (fig. 165, VI, VII), with obliteration of part or all of the intramural section of the tube, was in use by Johnson at Napa, by Traver at Patton, by Doan in the Pasadena General Hospital, by Weaver at Los Angeles, and by Prof. Frank Lynch at

From the book, Medical Essays by Medicus, 1931

Iatrogenesis: A Greek word which means "doctor-caused" or "doctor produced". It is a medical term meaning harm done by doctors, or negative side effect(s) caused by a medical treatment or procedure. The negative side effect(s) can be due to error, negligence, or can be caused by the standard protocol of the treatment.

Iatroepidemic: An epidemic of bad outcomes or negative side effects caused by doctors and their medical treatment(s) and procedures that become systematic. Examples of iatroepidemics include DES, and Post Tubal Ligation Syndrome (PTLS).

Diagnosed "627.2" "Post-Menopausal" Then "POF". My Quest for Support.

In 1995 I was in good health and was having regular cycles. For a means of birth control, my doctor suggested that I have a tubal ligation (TL). After my TL surgery my health changed drastically. I was not informed that one possible side effect of TL was menopause/POF due to ovarian isolation.

Two years later, at the age of 36 and in grave health my doctor ran blood work. My FSH was 92, and my LH was 27. At first I was literally told that I had "gone through the change of life" and was "definitely post-menopausal". When I met with my doctor two days later he told me that I was not post-menopausal, but "POF". I found this very confusing. Why was I told I was menopausal, and now was being told I was something else? I knew what menopause was, but didn't know what POF was.

I asked, "What is POF?" "Pre-mature Ovarian Failure" the doctor replied. I asked why I was not menopausal and he told me that only women over the age of 40 are diagnosed as menopausal and that women under the age of 40 are diagnosed POF. For "treatment" of my "POF" condition he gave me the birth-control pill.

I asked him if my menopausal/POF condition could have been caused by the TL and he told me, "no". However, a local Ob/Gyn told me that yes, it could.

I made my way to the Internet but could not find anything about "ovarian failure" or POF. I made contact with and joined the Sans Uteri group at www.findings.net. This is a support group for women who had hysterectomies. Although I still had my uterus and ovaries I related to this group because of the surgical menopausal syndrome everyone had experienced. The group's health concerns and postings were about treatment. My question was why wasn't it publicized that TL can cause POF?

Beth Tiner, the founder of Sans Uteri, suggested that I contact Catherine Corp, as she was forming an on-line group. I immediately contacted Catherine and joined the POF support group when it went on-line.

Like my experience at the Sans Uteri group, my experience at the POF support group was mixed. I was POF as the other women in the group were, but the majority of the women in this group were not POF due to ovarian isolation from tubal ligation or hysterectomy, but POF naturally or due to other means (such as chemotherapy or radiation therapy). Many women in the POF support were women who were diagnosed POF in their quest for becoming pregnant. Some women questioned why I was there. I had children and they did not. Their health concerns and postings were about fertility and treatment. My postings asked who was post-tubal and why women are not informed that tubal ligation can cause menopause/POF.

I gained a great deal of support and had a bond, yet I felt like an outsider.

I had a crash course on POF and menopause. I suffered being surgically POF (due to ovarian isolation, also known as surgical menopause or female castration) for two years with no HRT treatment. The menopause/POF I suffered was not natural but quite sudden and occurred quickly. I experienced hormone shock and then reverse shock when (proper) HRT treatment began. For legal reasons, I underwent a 2nd surgery to document the cause of my POF and found answers as to why women (and the public at large) are not informed of POF before tubal ligation surgery.

In 1998, with help and support from Dr. Vikki Hufnagel, the Coalition for Post Tubal Women came to be. The coalition's goals are to educate, inform, and provide accurate information to women considering tubal ligation; to educate, inform, assist, and create a supportive network for post tubal ligation women in their quest for answers and proper follow-up care, and to bring forth the needed changes that will require women to be fully and properly informed prior to tubal ligation surgery.

When the Coalition for Post Tubal began in 98', no medical or health related web sites spoke of post tubal ligation syndrome (PTLS), much less that tubal ligation can cause menopause or POF. Information about PTLS was not found in any type of information that explained tubal ligation. In the fall of 1999, the CPTwomen gained the support of the National Organization for Women (NOW) with the adoption of the "Tubal Ligation Resolution" which includes "educating the public".

With help from supportive men and women, doctors, and groups such as the POF support group, Sans Uteri, NOW, the media and press, and others, this information is slowly being presented to the public. Today a small handful of sites explain about PTLS and the menopause/POF risk and the numbers are growing. Unfortunately the American College of Obstetricians and Gynecologists still publicly denies that tubal ligation has menopause/POF risks. They allow and even encourage their members to withhold this information from women.

It has been interesting to see our progress, but our ultimate goal is to see all women informed of the menopause/POF risk before or at the time of consent to tubal ligation, not afterwards.

Dr. Hufnagel's actions of giving support to me, giving support to the Coalition for Post Tubal Women, and that of whistle blowing on a number of other issues has not been without backlash. What all has occurred to Dr. Hufnagel before and after I met her is a book in its self which is currently being written. What I can say is this; because of her courageous stance, someday all women will be properly informed and educated before any type of procedure which can affect their short or long term reproductive health.

Tubal Ligation IQ Test

1. Tubal ligation:

a. Is a form of permanent birth control.
b. Is labeled and promoted to women as a "band-aid" surgery.
c. In the US is in general always performed by an obgyn, ACOG doctor.
d. Carries risks which women are routinely not informed of at the time of consent.
e. All of the above

2. How many women have had a tubal ligation?

a. More than 1/2 of women age 25 or over
b. More then 1/4 of women aged 30 or over
c. More then 1/3 of women aged 18 or over

3. True or False:

"There is no risk that Tubal Ligation altering your hormonal system because it is not hormonal (as with the pill). "

4. True or False:
"Tubal Ligation is safe and without any known side effects (expect for the very small risk of pregnancy)."

5. True or False:
"Having a tubal ligation can improve the condition of endometriosis."

6. True or False:
"Having a tubal ligation can lessen your odds of getting ovarian cancer"

7. PTS is an acronym meaning:

a. Promote The Service
b. Profit The Surgeons
c. Post Tubal Syndrome

Answers are on next page

Tubal Ligation IQ Test: Answers

1. e

2. b

Tubal ligation is the most widely used form of birth control for women over the age of 30. It is estimated that between 750,000 to one million each year in the US alone undergo tubal ligation for the purpose of birth control and that 1/4 of all women of child bearing age world wide have been sterilized in some fashion.

3. False

Women are routinely NOT informed that there tubal ligation could possibly cause a hormonal imbalance that may require hormone replacement therapy (HRT) as treatment. The cause of a hormonal imbalance is veins, arteries, and capillaries (the blood supply) to the ovaries and uterus can and often are affected at the time of surgery. "Ovarian Isolation" (one or both ovaries being affected) happens because it is the nature of the surgery. The tubal ligation surgery does not have to be "botched" in order to experience ovarian isolation or some form of post tubal syndrome (PTS).

If both ovaries become isolated and fail it is the same as surgical menopause or female castration. This condition can cause hormone shock, bone loss, and other disabling effects such as loss of libido and sex drive, memory loss, confusion, out bursts of rage (uncontrollable PMS), hot flashes, and loss of balance. The few doctors who are currently willing to publicly comment on this event happening states that the risk of ovarian isolation is very low and not even worth mentioning.

Dr. Hufnagel states that the numbers of women who are affected by total castration (both ovaries affected) may be low, but that the numbers of women affected by some sort of PTS is more then 50%. The CPTwomen believes that the numbers are much higher then 50%.

4. False

There are 4 major categories of risk.

1. Surgical Risk: Infection, internal bleeding, complications from general anesthesia, etc...

2. Failed Tubal (Pregnancy) or Ectopic (Tubal) Pregnancy: Pregnancy after having had a tubal ligation can be serious because the risk of a tubal or ectopic pregnancy is much higher. If you are post tubal and believe that you

may be pregnant you need to be pregnancy tested right away. If it is found that you are pregnant your physician will need to immediately determine where the pregnancy is. If the pregnancy is located in your fallopian tube a surgery will be required as the condition is life threatening.

3. Tubal Regret: Some doctors screen to make sure that the woman has really put thought into their decision of permanent sterilization (meaning not able to have children or any more children ever). Other doctors don't (or don't care). The term "tubal regret" or "regret" has come to mean the woman regrets her tubal ligation because she now desires more children. We have termed this type of regret as "Baby Tubal Regret" (BTR). When a woman experiences BTR it is not really a surprise to her as she knows and understands the tubal ligation was the cause. Women are informed that the TL surgery is so that she can not have more children, she is not informed of the known side effects and risks which can lead to another type of regret which we have termed "Factual Tubal Regret" (FTR) which is explained below.

4. Post Tubal Syndrome (PTS) : Post tubal syndrome is the physical and physical effects which occurs caused by damage to the fallopian tubes, ovaries, and uterus and the effect of abrupt hormonal and physical changes caused by your routine tubal ligation or sterilization. "Ovarian Isolation", "Hormonal Imbalance", "Hormone Shock" and the "Cause and Effect" of the blood supply being altered to the ovaries and uterus are just a few of the "untold side effects".

Upon the realization of what the TL surgery did or might have done to one's health can also lead to "regret". This is not the regret of wishing that you could have more children but is regret, grief, sorrow, dread, horror, and dismay of learning that information and facts were withheld from you and that you were not informed by your trusted physician, and the regret of what the tubal ligation did to your health. We have termed this type of regret as "Factual Tubal Regret" (FTR), as this type of regret comes with learning the facts: the realization that information was withheld from you, that you were a victim of fraud and medical battery, and that you have been negatively altered or injured in some way.

5. False

There is no rhyme, reason, or evidence what so ever that tubal ligation improves or corrects endometriosis (unless the surgery is meant to cause you to become surgical menopausal.) When women enter menopause it has been noted that endometriosis becomes less severe. Surgical intervention such as Female Reconstruction Surgery (FRS) can correct endometriosis, but not tubal ligation.

6. True

The reason why this is true is never explained to women. The reason why this is true is because having a tubal ligation increases your odds of having a hysterectomy (at which time the ovaries would also be removed). Tubal ligation also can decrease or stop ovarian function, which in turn lessens the chance of ovarian cancer from developing.

7. c

Tubal ligations are known to cause a condition known and spoken of within the medical community as being Post Tubal Ligation Syndrome (PTLS or PTS). PTLS are the side effects caused by the tubal. As a unspoken code of silence, PTLS is not publicly spoken about by Ob/Gyn doctors, by the ACOG, nor are women informed of PTLS.

Causes and symptoms of PTS include:

   a. Hormonal imbalance caused by the blood supply to the ovaries being affected.
   b. The action of sealing the tubes can create a back flow/pressure into the tube (hydrosalpinx). The sealed tube(s) fills with fluid causing pain.
   c. Blood supply affected to the uterus can create the condition of andomyosis.

Women suffering from PTS often experience extreme heavy periods (gushing, flooding, cramping, pain). Causes include retro bleeding affecting the sealed tubes (hydrosalpinx), by areas of the uterus being affected by loss of blood supply causing theses areas to become atrophic, by a hormonal change (if the ovaries blood supply were affected) or by some of all.

Women are not informed of PTS at the time of consent, nor are they informed of it afterwards. Post Tubal Women are (as a matter of a canard obgyn, ACOG standard) are prescribed the pill (hormones) and told it is to "regulate their periods". This is done without first hormone testing.

Some women are told that told they are simply depressed, that their condition is mental and not physical and prescribed antidepressants (again these women are never hormone tested). Some women are sent to heart specialists because of menopausal effects such as heart palpation's. (again, never hormone tested). Many women with PTS are offered and suggested 2nd and 3rd surgeries such as D&C and hysterectomy.

Post Tubal Syndrome (PTS) Symptom List

Post tubal ligation syndrome (PTLS or PTS) is an iatrogenesis condition meaning doctor-caused or doctor produced. Many women suffer post tubal ligation syndrome after having a tubal ligation.

Post tubal ligation syndrome is often the result of a rapid decline of estrogen/progesterone hormone levels caused by the blood supply being damaged to the ovaries during the TL surgery. Depending on the damage to the veins and capillaries, blood volume to the ovaries may slightly decrease or can be eliminated completely which is called isolated ovarian syndrome (common with hysterectomy operations). Many of the symptoms of PTS are associated with menopause, hormone shock, or of having an estrogen/progesterone imbalance.

Other symptoms, such has heavy painful periods may be caused by a hormonal imbalance, could be caused by adenomyosis (bought on by uterus muscle and tissue being damaged, affected by the TL surgery impairing the blood supply to areas of that organ/muscle) or a combination of both. Pain also can be caused by retro bleeding backing into the sealed fallopian tubes causing a hydrosalpinx.

Other theories of PTS and the hormonal imbalance that results after a tubal ligation is that target or receptor cells that are important in the relay of hormonal messages are damaged, destroyed, and or removed as part of the surgery. These receptor cells act like a telephone, sending messages to the brain. These target/receptor cells are located within the fallopian tube. With this in mind, it's possible for a woman to have both her ovaries still functioning to some degree (if blood supply was not damaged), have no major problems with her uterus (again if blood supply was not damaged to that organ), and still be experiencing PTS in the from of a hormonal imbalance caused by a change in her hormonal message relay system due to receptor cells being removed.

The only way to find out for sure if you have a hormonal imbalance or are menopausal is to be properly hormone tested.

SYMPTOMS OF POST TUBAL SYNDROME

1. Etopic pregnancy or pregnancy (well known risk of tubal ligation)
2. Hot flashes, flushes, night sweats - cold flashes, clammy feeling, chills
3. Bouts of rapid heart beat
4. Irritability
5. Mood swings, sudden tears
6. Trouble sleeping through the night (with or without night sweats)
7. Irregular periods; shorter, lighter periods; heavier periods, flooding; phantom periods, shorter cycles, longer cycles
8. Loss of libido
9. Dry vagina
10. Itchy vagina-at time raw like, can radiated from whole area, with absence of yeast infections.
11. Color change in vaginal area. (color gets darker -darker red to purple)
12. Crashing fatigue - Chronic Fatigue Syndrome (CFS)
13. Anxiety, feeling ill at ease
14. Feelings of dread, apprehension, doom
15. Difficulty concentrating, disorientation, mental confusion
16. Disturbing memory lapses
17. Incontinence, especially upon sneezing, laughing; urge incontinence
18. Prolapse of uterus do to rapid decrease in estrogen levels.
19. Itchy, crawly skin
20. Aching, sore joints, muscles and tendons
21. Increased tension in muscles
22. Breast tenderness
23. Decrease in breast mass
24. Headache change: increase or decrease
25. Gastrointestinal distress, indigestion, flatulence, gas pain, nausea Irritable bowel syndrome (IBS)
26. Sudden bouts of bloat
27. Depression

28. Exacerbation of existing conditions
29. Allergies developing or increasing - (Chronic sinusitis).
30. Nasal infections-necessitating antibiotics
31. Weight gain
32. Hair loss or thinning, head, pubic, or whole body; increase in facial hair
33. Dizziness, light-headedness, episodes of loss of balance
34. Changes in body odor
35. Electric shock or stabbing sensation under the skin
36. Tingling in the extremities
37. Gum problems, increased bleeding
38. Burning tongue, burning roof of mouth, bad taste in mouth, change in breath odor
39. Osteoporosis (after several years)
40. Changes in fingernails: softer, crack or break easier
41. Stabbing pains in pelvic area at time of ovulation
42. Pelvic Pain
43. Development of Adenomyosis
44. Development of Ovarian/Tubal Cysts
45. Decreased Lactation Ability

The onset of PTLS is not always obvious to the post-tubal woman. She may know that she is sick and that she has suffered a health change but she may not always be properly diagnosed.

The symptoms of the hormonal imbalances that are often seen in post tubal women are often misdiagnosed by the medical community as being heart conditions, chronic fatigue, common depression, IBS, common allergies, and so on.

The medical community avoids hormone testing post tubal women under the age of 40. These women are told that they are too young to be post menopausal when in fact more often then not they are suffering from a hormonal imbalance or are post menopausal. Severe and prolonged hormonal imbalances of this nature can cause bone loss, heart disease, and can cause psychological symptoms that mimic mental illnesses and Alzheimer's.

NOTES:

Symptom 2 - (flashes) Hot flashes are due to the hypothalamic response to declining ovarian estrogen production. The declining estrogen state induces hypophysiotropic neurons in the arcuate nucleas of the hypothalamus to release gonadotropin-releasing hormone (GnRH) in a pulsatile fashion, which in turn stimulates release of luteinizing hormone (LH). Extremely high pulses of LH occur during the period of declining estrogen production. The LH has vasodilatory effects, which leads to flushing.

Symptom 8 - (loss of libido) For some women the loss is so great that they actually find sex repulsive, in much the same way as they felt before puberty. What hormones give, loss of hormones can take away.

Symptom 9 - (dry vagina) results in painful intercourse.

Symptom 10 - (Itchy and or raw vaginal area) A normal vaginal pH level is around 4.5. A vaginal pH of 6.0 to 7.5 -- in the absence of a vaginal infection (yeast infection)-- indicates low blood estrogen levels and signals that the woman is menopausal. "The vagina (and whole area) becomes more acidic."

Symptom 14 - (doom thoughts) includes thoughts of death, picturing one's own death. Feelings of complete despair.

Symptom 17 - (incontinence) reflects a general loss of smooth muscle tone.

Symptom 19 - (itchy, crawly skin) feeling of ants crawling under the skin, not just dry itchy skin.

Symptom 20 - (aching sore joints) may include such problems as carpal tunnel syndrome.

Symptom 27 - (depression) different from other depression, the inability to cope is overwhelming. There is a feeling of loss of self. Hormone therapy ameliorates the depression dramatically.

Symptom 31 - (weight gain) often around the waist and thighs, resulting in 'the disappearing waistline'

Symptom 35 - (shock sensation) This is often described as the feeling of a rubber band snapping in the layer of tissue between skin and muscle. It may be a precursor to a hot flash.

Symptom 36 - (tingling in extremities) can also be a symptom of B-12 deficiency, diabetes, alterations in the flexibility of blood vessels, or a depletion of potassium or calcium.

Symptom 38 - (Burning mouth syndrome)

Symptom 45 - Decreased Lactation Ability - This was reported upon in 1989 in Zentralbl Gynakol (111(16):1124-7) in an article titled, "The effect of postpartum tubal sterilization on milk production" by Vytiska-Binstorfer E. I. Universitats-Frauenklinik, Wien.

The study followed 64 women after tubal ligation and their milk production within the first seven days. They found that the total daily milk production, (which was compared with the quantity of milk after their previous pregnancies) was on days 6 and 7 significantly lower after tubal ligation than in the normal puerperal phase before.

Please note: Some of the symptoms above are also symptoms related to hypothyroidism, diabetes, iron deficiency, and other conditions. If you believe that you may be experiencing a hormonal imbalance or hormone shock, please contact your health care provider to consult and have proper serum testing done. Proper testing will check for ALL conditions. The findings of hypothyroidism, diabetes, or anemia does not rule out that a hormone imbalance is not also occurring. The findings of normal thyroid, insulin, and iron levels does not rule out that a hormone imbalance is not occurring.

"One of the most destructive things a woman can do to her body is to undergo sterilization. The sterilization process can cause damage and injury to women's reproductive and other vital organs in a number of ways." - Dr. VGH

Post Tubal Syndrome Examined

In medicine, the term *syndrome* is defined as a collection of health problems or symptoms that result from a single underlying cause that together form a condition with a known outcome, or which requires unique treatment.

Post Tubal Ligation Syndrome (PTLS) was first described by Dr. Vicki Hufnagel in 1980. She defined and reported on this syndrome to peer review medical associations. She outlined laboratory and diagnostic testing protocols to help diagnose the syndrome, created surgical repairs called Female Reconstructive Surgery for Post Tubal Ligation Syndrome (FRS/PTLS), and created medical treatments for PTS. She also wrote the first papers describing a need to change the informed consent to inform women about this condition. She has continued to provide the latest in clinical research and knowledge in the international health care arena for over 30 years. Dr. Hufnagel's clinical work has linked PTLS with the following:

- Castrative Menopause
- Severe Hormone Imbalance
- Ovarian Isolation (Post Hysterectomy, Post Tubal Ligation)
- Atrophic Ovaries
- Hormone Shock
- Increased Risk of Heart Disease
- Bone Loss and Osteoporosis
- Dysfunctional Uterine Bleeding (DUB)
- Pelvic Pain
- Hydrosalpinx
- PMS
- Atrophic Vaginitis
- Adenomyosis
- Severe Pelvic Adhesions
- Misplacement of Female Organs
- Decreased Lactating Ability

Castration cas·tra·tion

The term castration is commonly thought to be that of removing the male gonads (testicles) but the term relates to the removal or destruction of the primary sex organs (testes and ovaries) of either sex. Stedman's Medical Dictionary defines the term castration as something that can occur to the testicles or ovaries; sterilization. 1a.

Castration is any action, surgical or otherwise, by which a male or female loses the use of their testes or ovaries. When the testes or ovaries are removed or rendered non-functional, the person becomes sterile and the hormones that were produced by the sex gland (testosterone in males and estrogen in females) are no longer created or delivered.

In the 1700's and 1800's, young boys were castrated to persevere their high pitched singing voices for the arts. *Castrati* first appeared in the late sixteenth century in Spain, but the practice of castration to obtain fine voices took root mainly in Italy, where it remained until the mid-nineteenth century.

The castration of mature males historically was done to slaves and prisoners of war (torturing the enemy). Because ovaries are deep within women's bodies, historically women were not castrated as men have been. The castration of women has only been occurring with the development of modern medicine (surgery).

Medical Consequences of Castration

Ovariectomy, better known today as oophorectomy (female castration), is reported to have been first performed by Dr. Robert Battey of Rome, Georgia, in the late 1800's.

Concurrently, eugenics was being debated and supported by rich upper class to control the population of undesirables. Well-respected doctors began to promote the surgery for eugenic reasons and the surgery quickly became a popular medical fad.

Today ovaries are generally only removed in the case of cancer. The effects of castration upon young women have not been reported upon as that of the effects it has on young men.

Young males who are castrated before they begin puberty keep their high-pitched voices, delicate build, and small genitals. As they age they will not develop pubic hair and will have no sex drive or at best a very small sex drive. In history, there never was a time when pre-puberty girls were routinely castrated. Still, it is safe to say that the same effects would be seen in young girls with the addition that she would never begin to cycle or develop breasts.

The medical community calls a castrated man a "Castrate" (meaning that he was castrated). Today, castration is sometimes done as punishment (chemical sterilization of sex offenders), by men who undergo sex change operations, and as a treatment for men suffering prostrate cancer.

The following is reported by males who are castrated after the onset of puberty:

- reduced sex drive or no sex drive
- impotence and loss of erection
- erections take longer to occur
- The full erection does not get quite as firm as it used to
- Urge to ejaculate (organism) is not as insistent as before
- The force of ejaculation is not as strong as it once was.
- The amount of his ejaculate is less.
- The testicles shrink and the scrotal sack droops. The sack doesn't bunch up as much during arousal
- hot flushes and sweating
- Sleep disturbances, fatigue, muscle aches, stiff joints
- a rise in cholesterol with an associated increase in heart disease
- muscle mass, body strength, and bone mass decreases
- weight gain
- Feelings of Indecisiveness, anxiety and fear
- Feelings of Irritability and depression
- Loss of self-confidence and joy
- Loss of purpose and direction in life
- Feeling lonely, unattractive, and unloved
- Forgetfulness and difficulty concentrating, memory and concentration problems
- Taking longer to recover from injuries and illness
- Less endurance for physical activity
- The mature voice normally does not change
- Male balding does not occur, or stops if it already was occurring

It would be hard for an adult male who was castrated voluntarily or by force not to be depressed. Besides having lost his hormones and sex drive, he would be reminded of it every time he got dressed or when to the bathroom. It would be something that he could see was missing. Women who are castrated do not have a visual of the void. In all respects, a woman who is castrated looks pretty much the way she did before; expect she may have a scar on her stomach.

The term the medical community gives castrated women is not a castratee, but "menopause", or "surgical menopause".

Castration by Isolation

Dr. Hufnagel coined the medical term "ovarian isolation" and described the condition. While castration is most typically thought of the removing of the testicles/ovaries, it can also occur by isolating the organ from its blood supply. Being starved of blood, the organ is rendered useless and nonfunctional. Think of this as the organ being partially or fully detached so that it can be physically removed from the body, but then left inside. Castration by isolation can occur to both men and to women. The gland being without its blood supply shrinks becomes hard and atrophic.

The word atrophy is from the Greek meaning without life or void of life. Atrophic tissue is not found inside healthy human bodies. Atrophic tissue is only found were the blood supply was affected to the organ. (i.e., portions of brain can become atrophic after a stroke).

Ovarian isolation is a common side effect of hysterectomy (with saving the ovaries) and tubal ligation. The blood supply to one ovary, both ovaries, or neither ovary may be affected. If both ovaries are affected and become isolated at the time of a hysterectomy or tubal ligation, the loss of function of both ovaries constitutes a full surgical castration. If only one ovary is affected, it would constitute a partial castration.

In women, if one ovary is removed, or becomes non-functional due to ovarian isolation, a hormonal imbalance will occur. The remaining ovary does not begin to make twice as much estrogen as before and does not begin to release twice as many eggs as before. Some doctors have publicly stated that the remaining ovary would compensate for the loss of the other. There are no scientific studies that prove this and it defies all logic. Women who lose one ovary and still have their uterus often have irregular periods, some every other month.

If both ovaries become non-functional due to ovarian isolation in a pre-menopausal the sudden loss of estrogen will trigger an abrupt premature menopause. The sudden loss of hormones creates a hormone shock that may involve severe symptoms of hot flashes, chills, vaginal dryness, painful intercourse, loss of sex drive, and heart palpation's.

The medical community today usually informs women at the time of hysterectomy that if their ovaries are left in place they may fail, but they hold fast to their incongruous theory that ovaries are can not be affected by tubal ligation. The doctors who refuse to acknowledge PTS I believe suffer from another type of syndrome altogether, one that is yet to be named.

Hormone Shock

Some women after a tubal ligation develop dysfunctional uterine bleeding (DUB). DUB is a term used by the medical community meaning heavy or irregular menstrual bleeding that doesn't have any apparent underlying anatomical abnormality or cause.

While the condition of DUB can be debilitating, the effect of the loss of hormones can be equal to and even more damaging because of its effects on brain function, bone health, and heart health.

As women, we use estrogen in every cell of our body, including our brain cells. It makes us what we are. When both ovaries are removed or suddenly cease functioning, the sudden loss/stoppage of estrogen, hormones, and hormone shock can affect brain function. Confusion, rage, depression, and memory loss that can mimic an Alzheimer's type state can manifest. In addition to these symptoms, women who lose both ovaries, or lose the function of their ovaries, also lose the protection that these hormones provide against heart disease and osteoporosis many years earlier than if they had experienced natural menopause. Without treatment the symptoms and effects become greater over time.

Women who have had their ovaries removed or rendered nonfunctional due to ovarian isolation are seven times more likely to develop coronary heart disease and much more likely to develop bone problems at an early age than are pre-menopausal women whose ovaries are intact and functioning. The effects that it has on our brain function can not be measured but only reported upon.

Atrophic Vaginitis

Atrophic Vaginitis is a condition that is brought on by and aggravated by a sharp decline in estrogen levels. The cells in the vagina (12 layers of cells) thin out. What results is painful sex as there is less (or no) lubrication of the vagina. There is also less protection from vaginal infection.

In severe cases women experience dyspareunia, vaginal discharge, and a tight feeling in the vaginal area, but most likely several years after menopause.

Adenomyosis

Adenomyosis is one of the most destructive conditions of the uterus. The mainstream medical community states that there is no know cause as to why adenomyosis develops in women, and points out that it is rarely seen in women who have not had children, and this rarely seen in women under the age of 30.

Dr Hufnagel states the number one cause of adenomyosis is tubal ligation, hence why it is rarely seen in women who have not had children.

The standard routine treatment by US surgeons for adenomyosis is hysterectomy. Dr. Hufnagel, has pioneered several specific operations of import, including Female Reconstructive Surgery (FRS) for Adenomyectomy. FRS is an alternative to hysterectomy for the conditions of adenomyosis, hydrosalpinx, dysfunctional bleeding, endometriosis, and adhesions that can develop after tubal ligation.

Hydrosalpinx

A hydrosalpinx can occur anytime something happens to cause a fallopian tube to close. Fallopian tubes can close by injury or infection occurring to the end of the fallopian tube, the ampulla, and its delicate fingers, the fimbria, and by surgical means such as tubal ligation surgery. Glands within the tube produce a watery fluid that collects within the tube, producing a sausage shaped swelling that is characteristic of hydrosalpinx. Torsion can occur if the hydrosalpinx twists.

Tubal Spin:

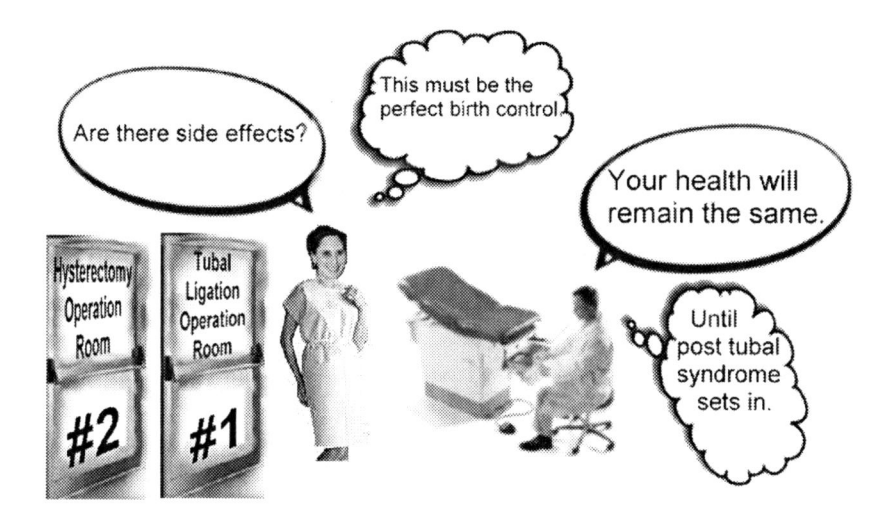

The obligation to disclose information rests on both ethical and legal foundations but ask any woman today what she was told of tubal ligation in advance and you'll learn that adverse outcomes such as ovarian isolation (causing ovarian failure/hormonal imbalance) and bleeding disorders leading to hysterectomy are never disclosed. - sjb

***The voluntary consent
of the human subject
is absolutely essential.***

- The Nuremberg Code

How Women are Diagnosed with Post Tubal Syndrome (PTS)

Post tubal syndrome (PTS): a negative health condition caused by side effects of tubal ligation/sterilization

The issue of information being withheld by the medical community has been compared to the large cigarette companies withholding information about the side effects of cigarette smoking. The only difference is when people got sick from smoking cigarettes they did not return to the same people who caused their condition and who withheld the information from them to start with. Their conditions were diagnosed.

Women suffering from PTS don't have a choice but to return to the same doctors and their peers that withheld the information from them to begin with. This gives the medical community a special power, the power to imprison.

Young women suffering from hormonal imbalances and pain caused by their tubal ligation are begging for help. They are asking doctors to help free them of their iatrogenic physical conditions but are denied an exit because the medical community that created their condition refuses to acknowledge that post tubal syndrome is real. - Susan J Bucher - 2003

The American College of Obstetricians and Gynecologists (ACOG) is the nation's and worlds leading group of professionals providing health care for women. The ACOG and their 40,000 obgyn members who perform tubal ligations KNOWS that there can be a sequel of negative effects to tubal ligation/sterilization surgery, AKA post tubal syndrome (PTS).

Doctors and researchers have spoken of, studied, examined and reported on this condition for decades. Published medical articles and studies show a direct correlation to tubal ligation and PTLS.

Although the ACOG is well aware that PTS is real, and that many peer reviewed, published scientific studies exist, the ACOG and their members withhold and deny the distribution of this information to women and the public. One way this information has been withheld is the medical/insurance diagnostic codes to describe/diagnose the PTS condition has never been put in place.

Coding is the transformation of verbal descriptions of disease, injury and procedures into numerical designations. Universally recognized coding systems provide information for reimbursement of health care claims, medical statistics and research. Literally every thing that happens within the medical setting from being given an aspirin, to surgery, to being diagnosed with a cold has a code assigned to it.

Dr. Vikki Hufnagel, (www.DrHufnagel.com) has been lobbying the ACOG and her peers for the past 25 years to get them to educate women about PTS and the true risks of tubal ligation/sterilization, and to put in place the proper medical codes which would allow physicians to officially diagnose women with PTS, or possible PTS.

Although PTS is well known there are no "official" medical/insurance codes assigned to the condition for physicians to diagnose a woman with PTS, or with possible PTS. This means that to date not one woman in the world has ever been officially diagnosed with PTS in the eyes of the AMA or the ACOG.

No official code puts a new spin on the term, "Code of Silence" (COS). The medical community's logic is if the medical/insurance code(s) do not exist, then the condition must not exist and no one could be diagnosed with that condition. There are no codes (nor plans for a code) because the ACOG with malicious intent misinforms the public and women that there is no such thing as PTLS, or negative side effects to tubal ligation/sterilization. The ACOG, our trusted women's health care providers, do not want PTS codes put in place.

The ACOG and their members have taken the deluded public stance that tubal ligation does not affect a woman's hormonal health, physical health, sexual health, lactating ability, bone health, or heart health. The ACOG states these falsifications to the public to protect themselves, their members, and their peers from the mass human and civil rights abuses they and their peers have committed against millions of women for decades.

The abuse is real & ongoing.

Physicians being trained to perform tubal ligations are directed to NOT inform women about PTS and of risk of negative side effects of tubal ligation. They are told that disclosing this information would cause the woman "conflict" at the time of consent. They are directed to report any and all health changes they see in post tubal women as that of "unrelated" to the tubal ligation.

The ACOG writes about "late sequelae" and promotes the denial of the known information with quotes and statements such as, "found little or no difference..., (follow-up) failed to identify a significant increase in risk...," and "risk has not been related..." (See exhibit #1 on page 61)

The ACOG promotes and adopts only the clinical studies that are formatted in such a way as to show little or no correlation. This allows them to promote TL as having no risk of PTLS, that PTLS is of no concern to women, and that women do not need to be informed or warned.

In this same technical bulletin, the ACOG specifically directs their members to state to women that there could be an "UNRELATED" change in their health. (See exhibit #2 on page 62)

Unrelated change is accepted by all women. All women accept that their bodies/female health will change as they get older. From the time we are little girls we are taught that our bodies will change and then we experience the change as our bodies develop and with the onset of menstruation. We also are taught that one day, if we live long enough, that we will also experience "The Change of Life", AKA menopause. Women accept the idea of unrelated or normal change, but not the ideas or facts of RELATED change due to a tubal ligation. It is the RELATED change in health that women need to be informed of.

OBGYNs do not make large sums of money doing pap smears, checking blood pressure, and prescribing pills... they make money by delivering babies and performing surgeries.

The ACOG and their members highly profit from tubal ligation surgeries. They profit by having themselves personally performed tubal ligation surgeries at some time, by teaching others how to perform tubal ligations, and/or by representing a strong lobbying group of doctors who perform and profit from tubal ligations and the common side effects which often manifest afterwards that will need future obgyn medical treatment and/or surgery.

The ACOG and their members are fully aware that tubal ligation surgeries can and often do create medical condition which will require women to return to the very same practice (obgyns) for medical attention. Most often these iatrogenesis (doctor caused) health conditions are resolved by surgical remedies such as D&C, and hysterectomy. The TL generates more business and money for their practice.

It is the ACOG and their members, not post tubal women (PTwomen) and their families, and not the authors and researchers who write and educated about PTS, who hold fast and make the public and private commits to women that PTS is not real.

The ACOGs standard of policy to not inform and to deny the risk of PTS is shown with the excluding of this information in the educational brochures they author and distribute. They put on a full persona that there is no serious short term or long term health risks or side effects.

"Sterilization by laparoscopy offers several benefits. A woman no longer needs to use birth control or to be concerned about becoming pregnant. It does not affect her menstrual cycle or sexual activity..." February 1996 Patient Education Pamphlet, developed under the direction of the committee on Patient Education of the ACOG. Distributed by the ACOG.   (See exhibit #3 on page 63)

10-14-1999:   NBC5 Chicago quoted the ACOG as stating, *"...the ACOG doesn't believe the syndrome is a medical condition..."*   To make their point NBC5 aired a taped interviewed of Dr. Serdar Bulun, M.D. (an ACOG member/spokes person) stating, *"so far there's no evidence ..."*

The ACOG states that, "there's no evidence ..." This is not true. There's much evidence and they are aware of it. The medical community has published many scientific peer-reviewed articles which show clear evidence of PTS. This information is provided to the public by the Freedom of Information Act.

The ACOG public denial of known facts, and their refusal to forewarn women of the known risks, and their direction, allowance, and support they give to their members and peers to withhold information has caused masses of women for decades to become a victim of this silent crime and to suffer with serious health conditions which the women themselves were not informed of or forewarned of.

Withholding known negative information with the intent to persuade the subject/patient to make a particular decision so that the one withholding the information will profit is medical and surgical fraud. It is also a criminal act of forced and coerced consent. To withhold information is a violation of human and civil rights.

Battery occurs when the woman has her body and health affected in ways which she did not consent to, and when she is injured unknowingly and with out forewarning.

The code of silence surrounding TL/Sterilization becomes more evident when it is seen how post tubal women (PTwomen) are treated when they return to their OBGYN physicians for help. PTwomen are discriminated against and denied hormone testing, diagnosis, and treatment, while young women who are not post tubal but are experiencing the same symptoms would be immediately hormone tested.

Hormone testing is basic for women. Physicians not hormone testing women having had a surgical procedure which is known to cause hormonal imbalances is causing more injuries and committing more batteries upon her if she is indeed suffering a severe hormonal imbalance/catastrophic menopause.

An untreated surgical menopause, or a severe hormonal imbalance, and the physical, mental, and sexual effects a women experiences with a the sudden stopping of hormones will not improve with time, but will become more devastating and more detrimental over time. The ACOG and their members know this information about untreated menopause and untreated severe hormonal imbalances. This is basic knowledge about women and women's health. The ACOG and their members also know that tubal ligation can cause hormonal imbalances of this nature.

Physicians also are well aware of and understand the rules and regulations of the COS. The COS which surrounds the issue of tubal ligation is so powerful that has its own COS, the "Tubal COS".

The doctor knows that no one is informed and believes she is still not informed. This compels the doctor to again give misinformation and to make statements such as "you're too young to be menopausal", "you do not have a hormonal imbalance," and "tubal ligations do not cause hormones levels to change". When physicians make these statements to PTwomen they make them as being absolute and undeniable.

Physicians who refuse to hormone test any woman who is experiencing a hormonal imbalance or a catastrophic menopause is in fact committing battery as well as the criminal action of forced imprisonment. The woman is imprisoned within her iatrogenesis health condition. If her condition is that of a hormonal imbalance, she could be freed from her negative health condition with proper testing, diagnosis's, and HRT treatment, but the doctor holds the key, and must open the door for this to happen. Only her physicians have the power to diagnose, prescribe, and treat.

OBGYNs are given the direction and peer support to not inform but must address the many PTwomen they routinely see in their practice. These women are truly suffering and they must be told or diagnosed with something.

Physicians are given health conditions such as Chronic Fatigue Syndrome (CFS), Depression (Stress, anxiety), Fibromyalgia, Irritable Bowel Syndrome (IBS), Dysfunctional uterine bleeding (DUB - cause unknown - unrelated to the Tubal ligation) etc.... to label or diagnose women with.

These are all health conditions which the AMA allows physicians to officially diagnose people with, (official codes have been put in place). These health conditions are not diagnosed with blood testing. The diagnosis is made by how long the condition persists, and the symptoms, and upon the doctors' opinion.

These health conditions (excluding depression) are primarily seen and diagnosed in women only. The symptoms of all these conditions match exactly what are seen in women suffering with severe hormonal imbalances such as which is found with untreated catastrophic menopause, or untreated female castration. In truth, many women who are diagnosed with these conditions may be suffering a severe hormonal imbalance, but the medical community does not test hormones to make the diagnostic decision to label women with these conditions.

Women who are diagnosed with conditions such as CFS, Fibromyalgia, IBS, dysfunctional uterine bleeding (DUB) and depression are quickly prescribed antidepressant, muscle relaxers, painkillers, etc.... These drugs may help a woman forget she's not feeling well, or help mask the pain, but will do nothing for the cause of her condition if she is suffering a severe hormonal imbalance. If she is indeed menopausal antidepressants and painkillers will not protect her against bone loss, developing heart disease, memory loss and her loss of sex drive that would be developing/occurring.

Many PTwomen are prescribed the birth control pill, and told that it is to regulate her periods, (if she is suffering DUB), but in fact the pill could cause the DUB to become worse which would cause her to be more likely to consider a hysterectomy. Doctors know that estrogen is the hormone which builds up the lining in your uterus. If you are experiencing heavy bleeding caused by an estrogen dominance, adding more estrogen is not going to correct.

The pill is also not appropriate for women needing HRT, and could cause the woman to stroke out if she is menopausal. For a doctor to prescribe the pill for a woman to be used as HRT or as a medical "treatment" (besides birth control), and doesn't give her the option or informs her of other safer forms of HRT is committing a criminal act of withholding information. If a woman is in need of HRT, there are much safer forms of HRT then the pill.

"Hormone testing before any form of HRT treatment is not an option, it's a necessity." - Dr. Vikki Hufnagel.

PTwomen seeking help and answers from their physicians regarding their current state of physical and hormonal health are immediately met with disallowance. Doctors are directed to not inform, and then dictated to never hormone test, otherwise the "Tubal COS" would be broken.

Think about it... if an obgyn in a community started hormone testing all PTwomen in his practice who were not feeling well, suddenly there'd be hundreds of young women within their practice/community all post tubal and all post menopausal. Word would get out not only to the PTwomen in the community, but more so to his peers. He would be breaking the "Code".

Breaking the COS is NOT to be done within the medical community. The doctor would be opening Pandora's Box. The most devastating wrath that would occur to his personal and professional life would be that which would waged upon him from his professional peers and superiors.

When post tubal women ask their physicians for hormone testing the doctors must decide whether or not to order the testing. The physicians literally weight their pros and con's on weather or not to help her and order the proper testing.

The PTwoman is discriminated against.

To hormone test could cause conflict for the doctor.

But then to not order the proper testing also causes conflict for the doctor.

The doctor must decide which the less of two evils is.

The tubal COS shows its true strength and power by the numbers of post tubal women who have who has been refused *proper hormone testing. Doctors rather abide by the tubal COS, then to help their patients. They rather be on good terms with their peers and avoid their wrath and punishment, then to submit to their personal and professional ethics, morals, and legal duties to their patients.

(*proper hormone testing is checking more then just one hormone level)

If the woman requests help or testing from the doctor who actually performed the TL on her he may feel as though he'd be exposing himself for having caused her the health condition. This causes even more conflict. If he wasn't the doctor who performed the tubal ligation, it's likely that he performs tubal ligations himself, and he might even personally know the TL doctor. The COS directs him to protect his peers. He would not want to expose a fellow obgyn, just as he wouldn't want a fellow obgyn to expose him. This is part of the all told code. The tubal COS with PTwomen is to never hormone test.

It's hard for PTwomen to accept that their doctors knew this information before their tubal ligation/sterilization and that their doctors withheld this information from them. It's even harder for women to accept that their physicians would refuse to help them now afterwards or to refuse to order proper hormone testing for them. The doctor clearly sees that she is suffering. This is a further demonstration how strong the tubal COS is, and brings more to the surface the horrendous crimes that have been committed upon women.

The ACOG and physicians who have performed tubal ligations have a full understanding of the true nature of the crimes that they have played out upon women. The tubal COS is much stronger then a code. It's directed to physicians by a medical Mafia style mentality and anyone who breaks the tubal code will regret doing so and will be made an example for others. Doctors fear breaking the tubal COS with good reason. When a medical professional breaks a COS they are submitted to personal and professionals attacks. Movies have been made about those who blew the whistle, or broke the code of silence. The insider, Erin Brockovich, and Karen Silkwood. Newspapers and magazines are dotted with stories about whistle blowers such as seen in the current Ladies Home Journal, January 2001, The Nurse Who Knew Too Much, page 94.

The size and magnitude of the tubal code, the shear numbers of violations and crimes which have occurred to women regarding TL/Sterilizations in the past century looms ivory towers over these stories. The tubal COS extends outside of the obgyn field and into other fields of medicine and has evolved and transformed to an altogether conspiracy.

Our Trusted Women's Health Care Providers ongoing actions of withholding this information are injurious, unethical, amoral, and criminal. It shows the ACOGs true regard for women, and their concern for the health and safety of the women that they are to protect and guide. They withhold this information in order to profit, at the health and expense of their patients.

The crimes that have been committed upon women regarding the withholding of this information are so scandalous, evil, and unjust that it's almost unbelievable. The numbers of women affected are too large to be believable. The whole historical effect can only be called an iatroepidemic female holocaust.

Because these issues of withholding information and cover-up exist, you will find it near impossible to find an ACOG obgyn, or any doctor to officially diagnose you in writing with having the condition (or possible condition) of PTS. Dr. Hufnagel is the only physician known by the Coalition who would do an honest review for a PTwoman and comment that her tubal ligation caused a post tubal ligation syndrome, or caused her current health condition if she thought or believed it to be true.

The majority of women who state that they are suffering PTS have self-diagnosed themselves. Women who suffer with PTS know it and don't have to be told or diagnosed. They know that they experienced a change in their health and can relate that change back to the time of their tubal ligation. A few women are softly and quietly verbally diagnosed with PTS by caring physicians, but these physicians would never put their diagnosis in writing for fear of breaking the tubal COS. PTwomen suffering PTS also know from first hand experience what the condition is, and that they were not informed or forewarned of PTS.

Mainstream doctors will never diagnosis anyone with the condition of PTS (or possible PTS) until the Code of Silence is removed, and the Diagnosis Medical Code created.

So what are the criteria for women diagnosed with PTS?

1. She had a tubal ligation, and

2. She had a sudden serious change in her health following the altering, separation, and or removal of some or all of her fallopian tubes.

Does this alone mean that a woman has PTS? Not necessarily but it does begin there. Some women report no health change after their TL. PTS is not easily diagnosed as all the injury/effects are internal and can not be easily seen.

To make a 100% sure diagnosis might require surgery to examine your organs and assess the damage that occurred. Biopsies of ovarian and uterine tissue could further make the diagnosis of PTS. With out this information a doctor might only state that it's possible that you are suffering PTS, and the degree of likelihood. As other health conditions are ruled out, and as diagnostic testing such as hormone analysis is done, the likely hood/possibility of PTS can increase.

Diagnostic blood testing can check for a hormone imbalance, ovarian function, and can rule out other conditions such as graves, auto immune, thyroid condition, etc... As conditions are ruled out the greater the odds are that there was an effect from the tubal ligation.

"There's only one way to know if a woman is experiencing a hormonal imbalance and that's to hormone test her. A doctor can not look at woman and make the statement or diagnosis that she not suffering or experiencing a hormonal imbalance. This is as absurd as a doctor stating they he could diagnosis people with AIDS by simply looking at them. Only proper blood testing can make this determination. Any doctor who states to a post tubal woman that they are too young to be menopausal, or that he knows without hormone testing her that she is not suffering a hormonal imbalance is committing medical fraud." - Dr. Vikki Hufnagel

Serum Hormone Analysis is mandatory for follow-up care of post tubal women and greatly aids women and their doctors in the diagnosis of PTS considering:

1. There is a risk that ovarian function could have been affected.

2. The hormone analysis can help determine ovarian function and diagnose a hormonal imbalance and menopause.

3. Menopause and severe hormonal imbalances of this nature are extremely rare in women under the age of 40. Young post tubal women finding they

have hormone levels in the menopausal range, (or experiencing a severe hormone imbalance), would be a strong suggestion that the tubal ligation had affected her ovarian function or hormone receptors.

So does/could serum hormone analysis alone diagnose the condition of PTS?

NO. There are other health conditions that the tubal ligation can create which may not affect hormones, such as adenomyosis or "atrophic endometrium." An atrophic, or ulcerated, endometrium can result when the blood supply is affected to areas of the uterus, and can also be caused by hormones. These causes (atrophic endometrium, severe hormonal imbalance) can in turn can cause the symptom of DUB.

Serum hormone analysis can help aid in diagnosing the condition of PTS, (to determine if ovarian function was altered/stopped) or the diagnosis may be that of a time line after your tubal ligation and atypical health conditions developing (such as dysfunctional uterine bleeding), how the condition progresses, the amount of time the condition persists, etc...

The time line for being diagnosed with PTS is not exact. Some women are immediately affected by their tubal ligation/sterilization and have symptoms suddenly develop shortly after surgery, (noted within the first few months to 2 years, etc..). Some women have symptoms slowly develop, (such as DUB), and the condition continues and escalates for 5 to 7 years (at which time surgeries such as D&C and hysterectomies are recommended).

Not all women develop PTS, severe PTS, or suffer all the symptoms of PTS or of a hormonal imbalance. Some women develop a minor hormonal imbalance, while others experience a surgical menopause/castration. Some women develop a hormonal imbalance but not DUB. Some women develop DUB, but not a hormonal imbalance. Some women experience both, and a few are lucky and are not affected all.

The Coalition of Post Tubal Women (www.Tubal.org) invites all women to register and join the Coalition in their efforts to educate women and create change.

"The most important thing is you and your health. If you believe that you are suffering PTS you must advocate for your own health first. Get hormone tested. Obtain copies of your medical records, labs results, and demand answers from your physician.... Register and become a member of the CPTwomen. The Coalition may be able to assist you. This is a grass roots effort. We must all work together to create the needed change." - Susan J Bucher - CPTwomen, Founder

Exhibit #1

Late Sequelae

The long-term health effects of tubal sterilization on menstrual pattern disturbance, pelvic pain, and the need for pelvic surgery are controversial. Early studies of menstrual disturbance following sterilization failed to account for confounding variables such as presterilization use of hormonal contraceptives that generally mask underlying menstrual dysfunction. Most recent prospective studies that account for these factors have found little or no difference in menstrual function between women before and after sterilization, or between sterilized women and nonsterilized control subjects in the first 2 years of follow up. Findings from reports that include follow up for more than 2 years have been less consistent, yet no single method of occlusion, regardless of the amount of tubal destruction, has been associated with an increase in risk for poststerilization menstrual disturbance (28).

Two studies have evaluated the likelihood of hospitalization for menstrual disorders in women who have undergone sterilization. A U.S. population-based cohort study showed an increased relative risk of 1.6 (95% confidence interval of 1.3–2.1) for hospitalization for menstrual disorders compared with a control group of wives of men who have had vasectomies (29). Follow up of a large British cohort for 6 years failed to identify a significant increase in risk (30).

Some sterilized women may be more likely to undergo subsequent hysterectomy. Women who have been sterilized before age 30 have a higher risk of a hysterectomy than women sterilized after age 30. This risk has not been related to an increase in menstrual disturbance or the extent of tissue damage based on the method of occlusion used (31).

Above: Late Sequelae information printed in the ACOGs Technical Bulletin, Number 222,-April 1996 - Sterilization

Exhibit #2

**ACOG TECHNICAL BULLETIN
NUMBER 222—APRIL 1996
STERILIZATION**

Components of Presterilization Counseling

Alternative methods available, including male sterilization

Reasons for choosing sterilization

Screening for risk indicators for regret

Details of the procedure, including anesthesia with attendant risks and benefits

The permanent nature of the procedure and information on reversal

The possibility of failure, including ectopic pregnancy

Post tubal ligation physiology, including the possibility of unrelated change in menstruation

The need to use condoms for protection against sexually transmitted diseases and human immunodeficiency virus infection if at risk of exposure

Answers to all questions to the satisfaction of the patient

Completion of informed consent document

Above: ACOGs "Components of Presterilization Counseling" directing their members to inform women of "unrelated" change to their menstruation.

Exhibit #3

> "Sterilization by laparoscopy offers several benefits. A woman no longer needs to use birth control or to be concerned about becoming pregnant. It does not affect her menstrual cycle or sexual activity..."
>
> February 1996 Patient Education Pamphlet, developed under the direction of the committee on Patient Education of the ACOG. Distributed by the ACOG.

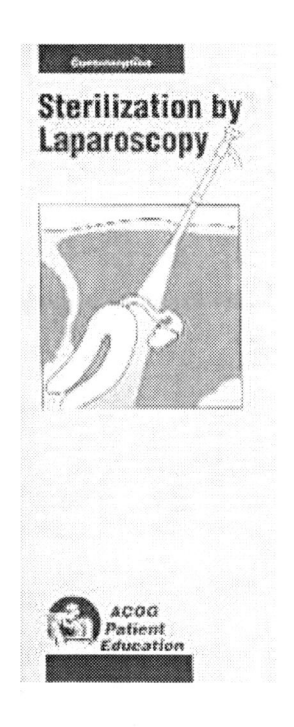

Case example #1 - Banding done 11-16-95

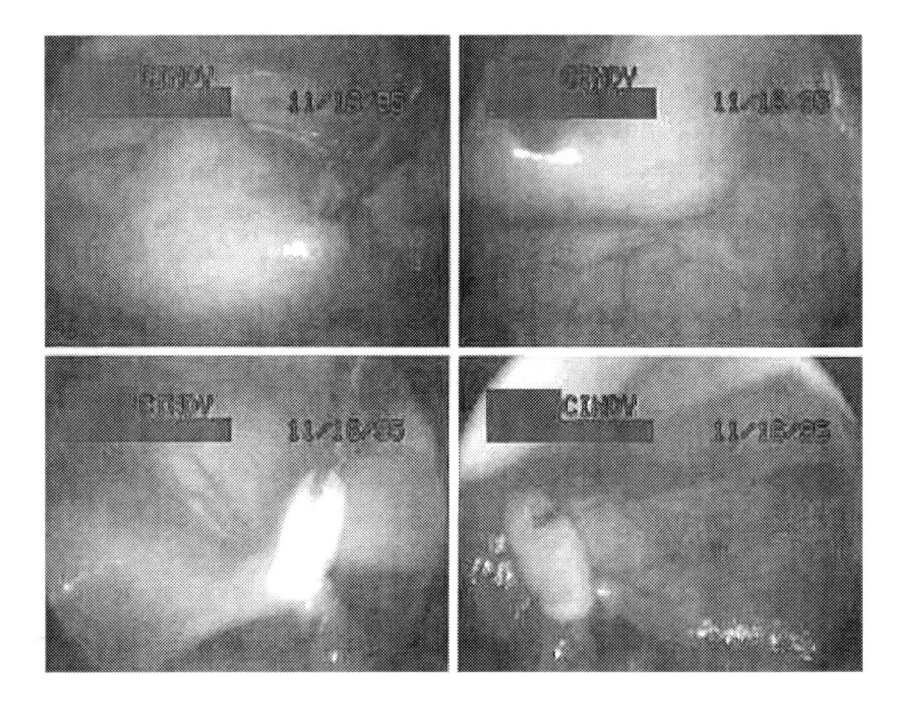

The above picture shows Cindy's fallopain tubes at the time of her "banding".

After this procedure, she suffered pain and irregular periods.
The photos on the next page shows the effects of this banding.

Effects of Banding

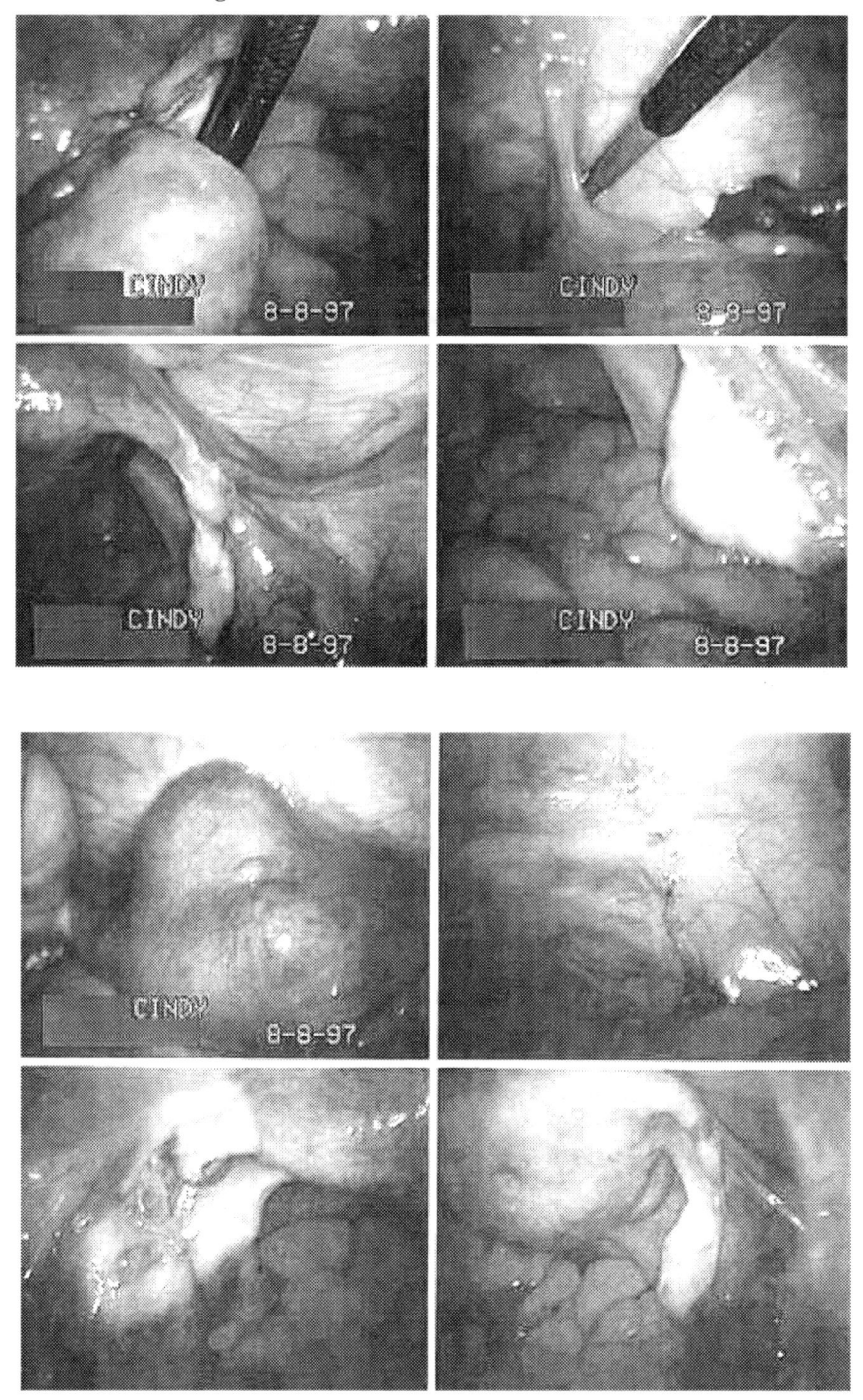

Case Example #2

Ovaries can become atrophic and shut down due to reuduced or eliminated blood supply.

This photo was taken on 8-24-95 at the time of a tubal ligation surgery. The blood supply was damaged which resulted in the ovary shutting down and becoming atrophic.

The 2nd photo is a photo of the same ovary on 7-21-98

3rd photo shows the other ovary (from the same woman) and how her other ovary appeared in 95'. The blood supply to this ovary was also damaged and this ovary also shut down and became atrophic due to the tubal ligation surgery.

4th photo shows how this ovary appeared on 7-21-98.

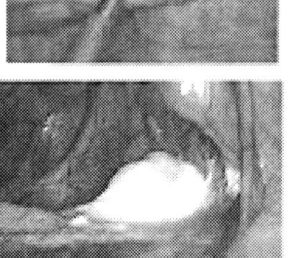

Losing one ovary to a tubal ligation surgery is more comman than losing both, but it does happen.
Tissue damage can also happen to the uterus due to altered blood flow.
Damage will happen were ever blood supply is cut.
If one or both ovaries survive, and tissue damage is done to uterine tissue, she may experince extreme periods.
Flooding and clots are commanly reported

c 1998

The fallopian tube is loaded with "receptor cells" which plays an important role in regulating your hormones. How much of your fallopian tube was removed at the time of your Tubal Ligation? - sjb

In the U.S., your odds are more then one in four of one day having a tubal ligation or hysterectomy. Your chance of one-day having a surgery that could affect your hormone production or possibly castrate you is much higher then getting breast cancer, yet women are not routinely offered hormone testing as they are with mammograms. - sjb

FAQ's about Hormone Testing
For Post Tubal Ligation Women

Q. Why should post tubal women be hormone tested?

A. Tubal ligations can cause ovarian isolation, catastrophic hormonal imbalances, castrative menopause, and hormone shock. The symptoms of menopause/hormone shock or that of a depleted hormonal state often first manifest as sleep disturbances/insomnia, chronic fatigue, hot flashes, depression, mood swings, memory loss, urinary infections/incontinence, and loss of sex drive. These symptoms and the condition of a depleted hormonal state can greatly affect a woman's well being, her social/work life, and family life.

Long term, a depleted hormonal state such as this if left untreated in a young woman can lead to accelerated bone loss, earlier and more severe cases of osteoporosis, and increased risk of and earlier onset of heart disease.

Q. What are the different types of hormone testing available?

A. Hormones can be measured using serum (blood), saliva, and over the counter (OTC) follicle stimulating hormone (FSH) test kits that work using urine. All three types of testing are explained here.

Q. Being post tubal, which type of testing is best for me?

A. Serum testing, but before you request serum testing from your doctor, you may want to start off by using an over the counter (OTC) home FSH test kit. These kits empowers and helps a woman determine in a timely manner if she is hormonally depleted, experiencing early menopause, or menopause, so that she can seek guidance and sound, appropriate advice/treatment from her personal physician. The usual reasons for constant elevated FSH levels throughout the cycle are related to menopause or the shutdown (failure) of the ovaries. Positive results from a home FSH test kit would absolutely merit further testing by your physician.

Q. How do the OTC home FSH test kits work?

A. These tests work like a home pregnancy tests. Urine is applied to activate the test. The results will indicate if the FSH levels are either over 25 mIU/ml (test reads positive) or less then 25 mIU/ml (test reads negative).

Q. Does it mean that I am menopausal if my test FSH is positive?

A. There is a short time during a menstruating (non-menopausal) woman's normal cycle when her FSH levels surge. This surge usually occurs mid-cycle. For this reason, the OTC FSH test kits are contain two tests so that in the event you do test positive you can re-check to see if your FSH levels remain evaluated.

The usual reasons for constant elevated FSH levels throughout the cycle are related to menopause or the gradual shutdown (failure) of the ovaries. As estrogen levels drop and diminish, the FSH levels rise. A positive test for elevated FSH (except at mid-cycle) is a clue to the onset of menopause or some other medical condition adversely effecting normal ovarian function.

Q. Should I request serum testing?

A. YES! The CPTwomen suggests that all women, including post tubal women, follow Dr. Hufnagel's outlined Base-line hormone testing and get serum tested.

Home FSH test kits are another tool that a woman can use to monitor her hormone health. These tests are less expensive that serum testing, does not require a doctors appointment, does not require travel to a lab to have a blood draw, and gives a woman accurate results in a matter of minutes in the privacy of her own home. Positive test results would absolutely merit further testing by your physician.

On the contrary, a negative test results does not mean that all your levels are in normal range. Your FSH levels could be just below the positive cut off. The home FSH test kits only measure FSH. The only way to know if your sex-binding hormone levels, thyroid levels, and other hormone levels are low or high is to be serum tested.

Q. I am 28 years old and had a tubal 2 years ago after the birth of my 3rd child. I do not think that I am suffering PTS, but have noticed that I am experiencing more intense PMS, intense itching (in the vagina area but I don't have a yeast infection), and have noticed a slight change in my periods. Should I be hormone tested?

A. Yes. All Post Tubal Women should get their hormone levels tested. Hormone testing for post tubal women should be standard care. Tubal ligations are know to cause castrative menopause, severe hormone imbalances, and PMS. The only way you can monitor your hormone health is to be tested. Surgical or sudden menopause is very serious and can cause the condition of "hormone shock". You could be experiencing a minor estrogen deficiency and experiencing slow bone loss with out even realizing that this is happening.

Vaginal itching is one symptom of having an estrogen deficiency.

Q. I am 31 years old and had a tubal ligation three years ago after the birth of my second son. I became extremely tired and fatigued and had had some dizzy spells so my doctor ordered some testing. I was told that all my levels were fine. That was one year ago. Now I'm having hot flashes. How can this be if all my levels are fine? I feel like I'm losing my mind!

A. For complaints of fatigue, it's common for doctors to order one or two tests. Generally only the TSH (thyroid stimulating hormone) and iron levels are checked. If your TSH came back came back normal that does not mean your estrogen, progesterone, SHBG, testosterone, FSH, LH, and other levels are normal. If your TSH comes back out of range, that too does not mean all your other levels are normal.

Women often told, "All your levels are fine", when in fact only the TSH and iron levels were checked. Women hear the word "all", and believe that all their levels were checked, and that no more testing is available or necessary.

Being post tubal you need to have the correct serum hormone testing done and you need to monitor your hormone levels. The doctor does not know how you feel, what you experience, and how you are functioning on a day to day basis. He is not going to be keeping track of your health, only you can do this.

Request a copy of the blood work that was done. You have a right to this information. Check and see what tests were ordered and what levels were checked. Where do your levels fall within the ranges? If hormone testing was done, it might be possible you were one or two points from being in a high/low range. Technically you may be within "normal range", but should be on an "alert" status.

If the correct basic hormone testing was ordered, and your levels were indeed within normal range then you will have this information as a base line and you should have the tests repeated in one year AND voice your concern now as to why you are not feeling up to par. One women early on with the CPTwomen went on for further testing and found out she had Lupus!

Q. What are the basic serum tests suggested a woman get?

Post Tubal Women-Hormone Health Protocol
*Indicates Basic Serum Testing

*Estrogen or Estradiol - test (E2)
*Progesterone (serum)
*SHBG - Sex hormone-binding globulin
*Testosterone
*FSH (follicle stimulating hormone)
LH (luteinizing hormone)
*Total Cholesterol. (HDL, LDL, and VLDL)
inhibin-a and inhibin-b
DHEA-sulfate dehydroepiandrosterone sulfate
Cortisol level
Prolactin (PRL)
Insulin
TSH - thyrotropin; thyroid stimulating hormone
Iron levels and B12
Note: When to test: For the best results and most optimum levels, blood draw for the estrogen, progesterone, and SHBG-Sex hormone-binding globulin levels should occur sometime in-between day 17 through day 20 of your cycle (day 1 being the first day of your last period). On these four days all of the female hormones are at high levels. If you are no longer having periods, or if you are having irregular cycles and are not able to determine when you had your last real/full cycle then it will have to be a guess. FSH levels, when checking to see if they are elevated, can be tested anytime expect for mid-cycle If FSH levels are evaluated or high in range, standard of practice is to re-check to confirm if FSH levels remain elevated. Some of the above listed blood work requires that you fast (no eating for at least twelve hours) prior to the blood draw. The <u>findings of hypothyroidism, diabetes, or anemia</u> does not rule out that a hormone imbalance or menopause is not also occurring. The <u>findings of normal thyroid, insulin, and iron levels</u> does not rule out that a hormone imbalance or menopause is not occurring. This medical protocol for Post Tubal Ligation Women was designed by Dr Vicki Hufnagel, MD

A. Provided here is the suggested basic testing. Not only should post tubal women get as a minimum the suggested testing, but it is advocated that ALL women should obtain these as baseline hormone levels starting at age thirty to thirty-five.

Baseline hormone testing for ALL women should be as standard as mammograms are for women at age forty. Loss of hormones or hormone production can affect both your physical and mental health (examples include bone health, memory, and libido). In the U.S., your odds are more then one in four of one day having a tubal ligation or hysterectomy. Your chance of one-day having a surgery that could affect your hormone production or possibly castrate you is much higher then getting breast cancer, yet women are not routinely offered hormone testing as they are with mammograms.

Having information about what your levels are when you are in the prime of your life and feeling your best is good information to have in your medical files if you ever need HRT or wish to match your baseline levels.

It is advocated that the following women should be hormone tested:

All women (including women younger then 30) should be hormone tested before all surgical procedures or medical treatments which could affect her hormone levels short term or long term: This would include being tested before a hysterectomy, tubal ligation, UAE, prior to donating eggs, lupron shots, and so on.

Women who are experiencing irregular periods or cycles. (regardless of age) This would include missing cycles (in absent of pregnancy), experiencing long periods (longer then 10 days of bleeding) long or short cycles (having two periods in a month, going 45 days between cycles).

All women who have had a tubal ligation, hysterectomy, UAE, one or both ovaries removed one or both fallopian tubes removed, or any type of surgical or medical treatment that could have affected her hormone production. (regardless of age)

Women who are suffering hormonal or menopausal symptoms such as: hot flashes, chills, night sweats, bouts of rapid heart beat, irritability, mood swings, trouble sleeping, loss of libido/sexual drive, crashing or chronic fatigue (CFS), anxiety, difficulty concentrating, fuzzy logic, memory lapses, sore joints/muscles, increase in headaches/migraines, depression, allergies developing or increasing, irritable bowel syndrome (IBS), sudden weight gain or loss, hair loss or thinning, episodes of dizziness or light-headedness, and loss of balance. (regardless of age)

Cholesterol levels start to rise as the hormones start to go, so women in menopause or experiencing a hormonal imbalance are at greater risk for heart disease.

Q. As a post tubal woman, is it important to have all the tests done?

A. YES. Measuring hormones and analyzing hormonal health is like putting together a puzzle. Many different levels are measured and then compared to each other. To check just one or two levels would be like looking at just one or two pieces of a 50-piece puzzle. Levels or measurements are grouped and analyzed in conjunction with others. For example, it would not make sense to look at a woman's FSH level with out also measuring her LH level. One is always compared to the other. Looking at only one of the levels would be like looking at only 1/2 of picture because you are getting only 1/2 of the information. Information from just one level is useless with out knowing the other level(s).

Q. I had a tubal ligation 5 years ago. Since then my periods have become very irregular. I believe I'm suffering a hormonal imbalance but my doctor told me that I'm too young to be menopausal (I'm only 34). He told me that I will not experience menopause until one year after my last period. He suggested to me a D&C to correct the bleeding disorder that I've developed.

A. First of all, if your symptoms (heavy bleeding) are being caused by a hormone imbalance, having a D&C will not correct (a hormone imbalance), it would only mask the symptom that is telling you something is wrong. Also, as was stated above, hormone testing should be done before any type of female reproductive surgery.

As women, we are taught that menopause is our periods stopping and ending. Some physicians state that a woman is not menopausal until she has gone for one full year without a period or bleeding.

Contrary to popular belief, your hormone levels (estrogen, progesterone, and testosterone) can be in the menopausal ranges and greatly depleted long before you experience your last period. To forgo testing (and therefore treatment) until one year has pasted with no period may mean one (or more) years of living with a condition which could be causing bone loss, increasing your risk of heart disease, and causing other physical and psychological changes. If you are a young woman and having a catastrophic menopause, the harder it may be to adjust your hormone levels later.

Irregular and heavy bleeding can be caused by and is one symptom of menopause, soon pending menopause, or hormonal imbalance. Irregular bleeding can also be a symptom of a tubal pregnancy, fibroids, and a number of other reasons, many which are not corrected by a D&C.

Your doctor can not say by simply looking at you if you are experiencing a hormonal imbalance or not, or if you are menopausal or not. Compare this to a doctor telling a patient that they don't have AIDS based simply by looking at them. The only way to know is to have the proper testing performed.

In the end, it may be a D&C which is required as your treatment, but wouldn't it be horrible to learn that you underwent a D&C only to find out later that it was a treatable hormonal imbalance?

Q. My doctor recently checked my levels (TSH and estrogen) and both came back normal. He told me that my levels are normal and that I am not suffering a hormonal imbalance. I do not understand how my hormones could be normal because I am still experiencing hot flashes and other hormonal symptoms. Why could this be?

A. A TSH test will not tell if you are menopausal or if you are suffering a hormonal condition but will diagnose a thyroid condition. It is possible to have a normal TSH level and to be suffering a severe hormonal imbalance (or to be post menopausal). Having your TSH checked is not a bad idea, but it is not going to tell you about your overall hormonal condition.

Analyzing just the estrogen level alone with out analyzing other levels is again like looking at just one piece of large puzzle. You are only seeing a small portion of the total.

It is possible to have your estrogen level come back in the normal range, but if your SHBG is low or high it could mean your estrogen deficient or dominant. It might have been that your estrogen levels were just one point away from being out of normal range. It is also possible to have normal estrogen levels but to have no progesterone which can greatly affect your health.

Your SHBG levels affect how much estrogen and testosterone your ovaries produces and how much is stored. If your SBHG level is high, low, or normal and comparing it to other hormone levels, and seeing if those levels are high, low, or normal gives a much clearer picture of your overall hormonal health.

High SHBG levels also plays a possible role in the development of endometriosis.

When analyzing hormone levels SHBG must also be analyzed. SHBG is key. SHBG should be routinely ordered every time your hormone levels are checked. If your doctor only ordered for you an estrogen test but no other levels hormone levels then your hormone testing was incomplete.

Q. What is the difference between blood testing, saliva testing, and the home FSH test kits?

A. Hormones are found in the system in two types of states, bound and unbound (free). Saliva testing measures the hormones that are unbound (free), or what is available for use at that very moment. Serum (blood) testing measures the total of both the bound and unbound (free). The home FSH test kits looks for unbound human follicle stimulating hormone (FSH) in your urine at a sensitivity cutoff level of 25 mIL/ml (anything less is negative, and thing more is positive). To compare the different types of testing is like comparing apples, oranges, and pears.

Serum hormone analysis has been and still is the industry standard, ordered and understood by all doctors.

There has been a big push by the manufactures and promoters of the saliva tests to sell, sell, and sell! Part of the marketing of these tests has been statements such as saliva tests are "more accurate" and "better". The truth is serum testing is accurate and is still the industry standard because saliva testing has limitations.

Saliva testing is good if you only want to know what is available for immediate use but bad if you want to know what your body is storing. Despite what some promoters of the saliva tests say serum testing is accurate, especially when the tests are grouped and ordered together so that they can be properly analyzed.

Q. Which type of testing is more accurate for testing estrogen and progesterone, the serum (blood testing) or saliva?

A. Serum analysis (blood test) measures the true total (100%) of both the unbound (free) hormones and the bound (stored) hormones. When serum tests are measured and analyzed it is known that 100% is the amount being analyzed.

The saliva testing and results can be greatly affected or altered by outside influences such as what you've recently eaten, drank, smoking, by use of the pill, hormone replacement therapy (HRT) and many other influences.

Measuring hormones by saliva does not measure 100% of all the hormones present but just the free, unbound hormones within your system. The amount of hormones that are free and unbound at any given moment is has been stated to be anywhere from 1% to 5% of the entire total so it's never really known if what is being measured is 1% of the total hormone present or 5 % of the total hormones present. Because it is known that serum testing measures 100% of the total this makes the serum testing a more exact measurement because there are no unknown variables.

Because the saliva testing measures the amounts what your body can actually use at that moment it has been strongly inferred and often outright stated by the promoters of these tests that the saliva testing is better then serum testing. Women have been told, "what's the point of knowing how much hormones you're storing, you can't use them anyway so what's the point?" Women are told that, "it doesn't matter how much is being stored..." Yes, women have been told that this information is not necessary! Saliva testing is can measure what is free and unbound but to infer because saliva can make this measurement that it's better then serum at determining a woman's overall hormonal health is just not true.

A comparison could be made to fat and energy. We have energy stored in fat as calories. Energy is continuously available to us (we even burn calories when we sleep.)

A small portion of energy is always available for immediate use and the rest is stored. To tell a woman how much "energy" she has at any given moment, or how many calories she is currently burning but then to tell her that it doesn't matter how much she weighs, that it doesn't matter what percentage of her body weight is fat, or to make statements that it is not necessary to know this information for good health would be inaccurate. The same goes for hormones. When analyzing a women's hormonal health it is very important to know how much is being stored and in what levels.

Only serum analysis (a blood test) can measure SEX BINDING HORMONE (SHBG) because saliva testing can not measure proteins. Do not get confused that SHBG is a hormone because of the word hormone is in its title. SHBG is not a hormone. SHBG is a protein. SHBG is the principle protein that regulates and binds hormones together leaving just a small percentage (1% to 5%) free and unbound. Saliva testing only measures hormones, it can not measure proteins. You can spit out hormones but you cannot spit out proteins.

SHBG levels can determine if your hormones are being bound and in what amounts. Your SHBG levels also affect how much estrogen and testosterone your ovaries produces. If your SBHG level is high, low or normal and comparing it to your hormone levels, and seeing if those levels are high, low, or normal gives a much clearer picture of your overall hormonal health then saliva testing.

Q. So is serum hormone analysis better then saliva testing?

A. Both types of tests are good at what they do. They both look for the same thing (hormones) but in different forms.

For applications such as obtaining baseline levels and yearly monitoring the serum testing is better. Saliva testing is good for other applications such as women under going fertility treatments, and the home FSH test kits have a place in women's healthcare as well. Women at times might choose to all types of testing in combination.

For anyone to state that one type of testing is better then the other, or that saliva testing is the only testing women need is wrong. Each type of testing has their place and role in the arena of women's health care.

Q. How does the home FSH test kits compare to the serum and saliva testing?

A. The home FSH test kits are very good at what they do. They measure and detect human follicle stimulating hormone (FSH) in urine at a sensitivity cutoff level of 25 mIL/ml (anything less the test reads negative, anything more the test reads positive). The usual reasons for constant elevated FSH levels throughout the cycle are related to menopause or the gradual shutdown (failure) of the ovaries.

In order for your FSH levels to be constantly evaluated, other hormone levels (i.e., estrogen) first need to be low (in the menopausal range). Consequently, a positive test for elevated FSH (except at mid-cycle) is a clue to the onset of menopause or some other medical condition adversely effecting normal ovarian function.

A positive qualitative test for elevated levels of FSH does not, under any circumstance, confirm or deny a diagnosis of menopause or ovarian failure. If you do home testing such as this and have positive test results, further tests and consultation with a healthcare professional are required.

Q. What if I get serum hormone tested and all my levels are normal?

A. If your levels are in normal range the information will provide you with a baseline for future reference. If they are not in normal range you may want to consider therapy options.

FYI. Hormones act on their target cells by way of receptors: specific sites on or inside the cell bond with the incoming hormone and initiate the cell's response to the hormone. Feedback loops often involve changes in the receptor content of target cells; an increased or decreased receptor content results in increased or decreased responsiveness of the cell to any given level of incoming hormone.

The fallopian tube is loaded with "receptor cells" which plays an important role in regulating your hormones. How much of your fallopian tube was removed at the time of your Tubal Ligation?

Do Doctors Steal Eggs?

When I first learned that I was postmenopausal in 1997, having been told by Dr. PC that Dr. R probably caused my condition by cutting my ovarian arteries during my tubal ligation surgery, I began to research on the Internet. I could not comprehend that this was a common risk, and even more incomprehensible, was the fact that I hadn't been forewarned of it. I wanted to see were I missed this information. I wanted to learn what occurred at the time of my surgery that caused my ovaries to fail, and what things in general causes ovarian failure.

To begin with I couldn't find any information about side effects to tubal ligation. All the sites that I visited that mentioned tubal ligation were medical sites/clinics that offered the service. Eventually, my search lead me to GratefulMed (now known as pubmed.gov). Besides finding articles about tubal ligation, I also found articles about ovaries being adversely affected from chemotherapy, radiation, and ovarian torsion.

Torsion, I learned, is a condition in which an enlarged ovary twists or turns on its supporting ligament, causing great pain and cutting off its blood supply. Torsion can be caused by an ovarian cyst. It is also risk for women who donate eggs for In Vitro Fertilization (IVF) use because they are given hormones/drugs such as chorionic gonadotrophin to "hyper-stimulate" their ovaries to cause a super-ovulation (the release of several eggs in a single cycle). This causes the ovaries to enlarge sometimes as large a grapefruits. I thought, "O.K., this isn't me because I didn't take drugs to hyper-stimulate my ovaries, I didn't have pain episodes, chemotherapy or radiation treatments…" Then a flush came over me. Could it be possible for a doctor to take eggs at the time of a tubal ligation without the woman knowing and without being given drugs to hyper-stimulate their ovaries and then sell the eggs as being "donated"?

The answer is "yes".

In Vitro Fertilization (IVF) is primarily used to overcome female infertility. The first test tube baby in the US was born in 1981. Since then, there have been remarkable advances in human reproductive technology. IVF today is a highly lucrative market and is largely privately funded and almost completely unregulated.

The concept of IVF is elementary; a ripe human egg (called an oocyte) is extracted from the ovary shortly before it would be released and is mixed with semen so that fertilization can occur. The fertilized egg is then transferred back to the mother's uterus or fallopian tube.

In the early days of IVF, during egg collection, doctors and scientists didn't manipulate the ovaries with hormones but would harvest a single egg during a woman's natural cycle. The doctors were faced with the problems of having to carefully time the harvest of the egg. Typically, oocytes mature only a few hours before ovulation and it was very difficult to collect an oocyte that was matured or "ripe". If their timing was off and they were too early the egg would not be mature and it would not fertilize. If they were late in retrieving the egg is would be lost within the body.

The process of harvesting eggs from a womans' natural cycle was very involved and costly. The women was required to undergo stringent monitoring such as having her blood drawn every 2-3 hours, and IVF teams had to be ready round the clock to perform the egg retrieval at the optimal time. Because only one egg could be collected at during each cycle, women undergoing IVF often would often undergo monthly these costly, invasive, not to mention emotionally draining procedures in search of a single egg to fertilize. In addition, each procedure carried with it the usual risks of surgery, such as infection and risks associated with undergoing anesthesia. Even if an egg was collected, that didn't mean that the egg would become fertilized and work.

In time, IVF evolved as women were able to donate eggs to other women desiring babies. Doctors sought ways to collect multiple eggs at the time of a harvest. They learned that that by using hormones they could "hyper-stimulate" the ovaries. This was a big advance for the industry. More eggs at each retrieval meant better odds that women would have a successful IVF treatment. It also meant more eggs for study and to be donated to other women. As quickly as this happened, the supply of eggs was severely curtailed because cryopreservation was made available. Women, instead of donating their extra eggs to other women or research were choosing instead to save their harvested eggs for future personal use.

With cryopreservation and the sudden decline of women donating all their unused oocytes for altruistic reasons, Doctors needed to find other sources of eggs for their clients. Doctors began to advertise for egg donors (mostly on college campuses) for anonymous donors who would be paid a fee. Doctors also saw women undergoing laparoscopic serialization as a possible source of eggs. In 1987, the Women's Medical Pavilion in Dobbs Ferry, New York conducted a study to learn the willingness of women undergoing a tubal ligation in donating eggs. Their findings were that tubal ligation patients where unwilling to donate oocytes despite "enthusiastic counseling", and their offers of financial compensation.

The IVF community from the start shaped the doctrine that all egg donations should remain anonymous. They also created the policy that the recipient of the egg(s) would be charged a fee that would be passed back to the donor to "compensation" or "reimbursement" for the donors time and effort. The IVF industry being unregulated, their practice of keeping egg donations anonymous, and the huge demand for eggs that could be sold for profit quickly created a black market. Couples and research labs that paid for eggs had no way of knowing if the eggs were truly donated. Often it was said the eggs were donated by a woman who gave "verbal" consent.

Dr. Ricardo Asch and Dr. Jose Balmaceda formally associated with the University of California, Irvine, (UCI) Center for Reproductive Heath, were two doctors that cashed in on the opportunity that was presented to them in the 80's and 90's. They sold harvested eggs, which were supposed to have banked, without the knowledge or permission of their patients, to unsuspecting infertile couples and research labs under the guise that they had been donated.

As this "fertility scandal" erupted, the university closed its center and Asch and Balmaceda fled the country. Susan Kelleher, in 1995 while working for the Orange County Register, won a Pulitzer Prize for her reporting of this story. Ultimately, UCI paid over 20 million dollars to settle the one hundred and thirteen suits lawsuits that were brought against them.

Although this case occurred over 10 years ago, it is still making front page news. On January 20, 2006, the LA Times reported, "When revelations surfaced a decade ago that fertility doctors at UCI Medical Center had stolen eggs and embryos from patients, the university vowed to find the women who may have been victims. But UC Irvine acknowledged this week that it failed to contact at least 20 couples, some of whom have learned only in recent years that their fertilized embryos produced children born to other women more than 15 years ago." www.latimes.com

As a result of the UCI scandal, California became the first state to have a law that explicitly recognizes egg donation. It requires that donors provide explicit informed consent, as well as specify how they want unused donated material to be handled. Doctors who fail to obtain proper consent (if they are caught) can be slapped on the wrist with a fined up to $5,000.

Still, Drs. Asch and Balamceda were not the only doctors in the US involved in the study and service of human reproduction, and UCI's Center for Reproductive Heath was not the only fertility clinic in the US. I believe that Asch and Balamceda fleeing the country was twofold. One was to protect themselves from going to jail, but second was to protect others from being implemented.

Asch had contacts throughout the US. One doctor who was tied to Asch, Dr. Gerald Schatten had, while associated with the University of

Wisconsin in 1990, purchased and used several hundred eggs from Asch. Schatten escaped persecution as he stated that he believed that the eggs were knowingly donated, and that he had been "duped". Today Schatten is a Pennsylvania-based stem cell researcher.

The UCI fertility scandal, while highly publicized, was not an isolated case. Since 1995, reports of misdoing have repeatedly surfaced regarding doctors and clinics from New York to Hawaii. The temptation for doctors to take unused eggs and present them as being donated, while collecting (and keeping) a fee that is thought to be passed back to a donor, still presents itself.

How far wide spread the black market is, or will evolve to be, is only a guess. One thing is clear, the supply for human eggs today is greater then it's ever been, and the demand just grew larger with the passage of Proposition 71 that created The California Institute for Regenerative Medicine (CIRM). . The CIRM is mandated to progress and prioritize stem cell research and was given $3 billion to be used and distributed to facilities. http://www.cirm.ca.gov/

The goal of the CIRM is to develop using genetic engineering cures to human diseases, ranging from Huntingtons to cancer. In order to do this the CIRM and researchers are going to need human eggs, hundreds and thousands of them. Where are all these eggs going to come from?

It has been proposed that these eggs be obtained from women at the time of tubal ligation, and that the best and safest way would be to extract the eggs with natural cycling (involving no hormonal manipulations of the ovary).

While obtaining oocytes during a natural cycle was once very difficult, it is easily and routinely done today because matured eggs can be obtained from women's ovaries, placed in some follicular fluid and ripened. Study in immature oocyte retrieval, maturing of the egg, fertilization, and implanting has been studied and successfully practiced since at least 1991.

The process of collecting immature eggs is as easy as drawing blood. Using a needle, immature eggs are collected directly into a small vacuum sealed test tube. The eggs are mixed with a follicular growth fluid and the eggs mature. Once mature, the eggs can be used right away, or they can be frozen for future use. Multiple immature eggs can be collected and brought to maturity at each harvest and the number of eggs obtained is comparative to harvesting eggs from an ovary that is hyper-stimulated. The immature eggs can be harvested directly from the ovary, or from ovary tissue (a section of ovary) that has been surgically removed.

While it's illegal to sell any human body parts, it's not illegal to sell eggs. Human eggs go to the highest bidder. Today the American Society for Reproductive Medicine recommends that women who donate eggs for fertility purposes be paid between $5,000 and $10,000. Knowing the value of an egg, and how easy it would be to obtain eggs at the time of tubal ligation, I suspect that there may be doctors today who harvest eggs during tubal ligations, mature them, and then sell them on the black market as having been donated. This would be very easy and profitable for doctors as they would pocket the fee meant to be used to compensate the donor.

Doctors doing this might have the attitude that "hey, she's having a tubal ligation, she doesn't want more kids, she's never going to use these eggs, she'll never miss these eggs".

The following letter was posted at tubal.org and caught my attention because she suffered "a cut to both ovaries".

It is nice to know I am not alone

by Christine - Posted on Jun 27, 2001, 10:12 AM

I had a TL on April 4 2001, my doctor told me that the very next day I would be feeling 75% better and could resume normal activities. I wish that had been the case, I actually felt worse and the pain from the simple "band aid" surgery was unbelievable. Several calls to the doctor's office later I was told that it was simple post surgery pain and that I needed to keep resting....(what happened to 75% improvement??). 8 days later I ended up in ER with what they now know was peritonitis, **a cut to both ovaries...**

Recently I came across an article titled, "Who Are the Women Who Donate Oocytes?" at www.dentalplans.com/Dental-Health-Articles/Oocyte-Donation.asp. It states that besides getting eggs from known donors (such as a sister, other relative, or friend) and anonymous donors, that some centers recruit women undergoing tubal ligation(s) to donate oocytes. When I underwent my tubal ligation in 1995 I was not asked if I wanted to donate eggs. In talking to thousands of women the past 10 years, no one has ever told me that they were asked to donate eggs at the time of their tubal ligation. I wonder what doctors and which centers these are that are recruiting women. Are they really asking women if they would like to donate eggs? I question how many women have eggs taken during a tubal ligation without them knowing.

My purpose in presenting this information is not to suggest that I or anyone has been a victim of having eggs harvested at the time of tubal ligation, which were then sold on the black market. It is to open a debate and to bring awareness that it's possible for this to occur, and to further demonstrate the need for informed consent and monitoring of doctors who perform tubal ligation and who work in the sector of human reproductive sciences.

One debate the CIRM has created is weather or not women should be compensated for donating eggs for this newly created Stem Cell Research program. They have a theory that offering compensation for donated eggs would create a black market and lead to corruption and abuse. I believe that the black market and corruption already exists, and will continue until changes are made and laws put in place to protect the rights of women.

For more history and perspectives on the above issues regarding IVF, stem cell research and abusive in this arena, I suggest the following Internet links:

brown.edu/Courses/BI0032/IVF/a.html

californiastemcellreport.blogspot.com/2005_03_01_californiastemcellreport_archive.html

cincinnatifertility.com/In_Vitro/Full_Text_Article.htm

cirm.ca.gov

drmalpani.com/darkside.htm

etopiamedia.net/empnn/pages/cpt-emnn/cpt-emnn470-5551212.html

genetics-and-society.org/policies/california/

genetics-and-society.org/resources/background/eefactsheet.html

genetics-and-society.org/resources/cgs/20050307_cirm_press.html

ivf.co.il/egloss.htm

ivfneedles.com/ product.php3?gid=240

mpssociety.org/leg-res-research1.html

pbs.org/bloodlines/timeline/text_timeline.html

pubmed.gov

spuc.org.uk/ethics/art/

The Magic Cure to Post Tubal Syndrome

Post Tubal Ligation Syndrome: Iatrogenesis affects that create negative health conditions after a tubal ligation or female sterilization surgery. Can be hormonal and or physical in nature. Health changes both physical and hormonal can cause mental health to be affected, causing loss of sexual drive for the woman, memory loss, depression, anger and rage. Physical effects include pelvic pain and bleeding, which often results in surgical treatments.

"Hysterectomy is NOT a cure for PTS and just putting the tubes back together does NOT fix all the things that go wrong after a tubal ligation. The pathology I find in about 80% of post-tubal women is andomyosis (which causes pain and bleeding disorders) and adhesions. Tubal reversal does not fix a hormonal imbalance, does not correct pelvic adhesions, and does not correct andomyosis.

- Dr. Hufnagel,

    To date I can not think of a single thing that cures any disease or condition. There are only treatments. The Coalition is often asked, "Will a reversal help me? Will a reversal reverse my symptoms?"

    My reply is, "How does one reverse something that is irreversible? How does one replace fallopian tube and receptors cells that have been removed or destroyed? Compare it to undoing a lobotomy."

    The first question I ask is their reason for a reversal so you can go on and have more children, or is it being done to reverse negative health symptoms? If the reversal operation is being done to reverse negative health symptoms, then it really isn't a reversal because the medical community and the insurance companies view a tubal reversal as a surgery that is done in attempt to restore fertility, not to relieve pain, correct a bleeding disorder, restore blood supply and hormone production.

    A reversal surgery is just putting the fallopian tubes back together. It does not address the conditions found in women with post tubal syndrome such as adhesions, andomyosis, ovarian/fallopian cysts, compromised blood supply, atrophic tissue, and other pathology.

    One problem noted with all the doctors that do reversals is that they do not hormone test before a reversal. Why is that? They may ask women for copies of their medical records from their tubal ligation, and women will have standard pre-surgical blood work and tests done, but they are not tested for menopause to see if their ovaries are even functioning. What good is a reversal to restore fertility if your ovaries are not producing eggs?

Women suffering from post tubal syndrome seeking a cure to their condition are often lured into the idea that a reversal is going to help them and "reverse" their negative health symptoms. The word "reverse" in the word "tubal reversal", does not apply to reversing PTS.

The truth is women who do NOT have symptoms of PTS and were not affected by their tubal ligation are more likely to have a successful reversal and go on to have more children then those who were affected by their tubal ligation and who are experiencing symptoms of PTS.

Still, if you've had a tubal ligation, you will have no problem finding a "tubal reversal" doctor will take your money and perform a surgery that's meant to restore your fertility without first checking ovarian status. The reason ovarian status is not checked before a reversal surgery is because if the doctor knew in advance that the woman has no ovarian function then it would be meaningless for the doctor to perform the surgery. The doctor would have to disclose to the woman that "even if" there were enough tube to connect a pregnancy would not result because her ovaries no longer producing and releasing eggs. Telling the woman this the surgeon would most likely lose a sale, hence why ovarian function is not evaluated before a tubal reversal.

If one is seeking medical care regarding the condition of post tubal syndrome, it's not a reversal surgery that they are looking for. Unfortunately, D&C's, ablation, and hysterectomies are the treatments suggested to women suffering post tubal syndrome, not hormone testing to diagnose/treat a hormone imbalance or FRS (corrective surgery) to save/reconstruct organs.

Dr. Hufnagel's Female Reconstructive Surgery (FRS) is an alternative to tubal reversal or hysterectomy for post tubal women suffering pain, bleeding disorders, and other effects of PTLS. Tubal reversal surgery simply does not address these symptoms.

While some women may opt to try for a surgical remedy to their PTLS condition, the true cure to PTLS would be that of informing women of the risk of PTLS before they consent to the surgery.

About the Coalition for Post Tubal Women

The CPTwomen is non-partisan, non-denomination, and most of all we are NOT anti-tubal. We believe that tubal ligations should be made a choice to women as a form of birth control but with FULL consent.

Tubal ligation is a surgical procedure done for permanent birth control. It is promoted by the American Medical Association (AMA), the American College of Obstetrics and Gynecology (ACOG) and by obgyns who perform the surgery as being without known serious side effects, but this is NOT true.

Post Tubal Syndrome (PTS) has been medically proven to really exist. We ask why women were not and are still not being informed?

What we are is anti-doctors/ACOG withholding information from women in order to force the women's consent. Information is withheld to persuade women to make the decision that the doctor wants them to make. Withholding negative information from women at the time of consent is an intentional fraud. Doctors and organizations who state there are no side effects to tubal ligation are committing intentional fraud and misrepresentation

The issue is "Informed Consent" because information IS being withheld. The action of withholding this information is a crime. The crime is fraud which overlaps to assault.

This fraud and assault is creating a "hormonal iatroepidemic holocaust" which will one day, very soon, be exposed as one of the most shocking "medical cover-up crimes of the century".

Repeatedly we hear women stating,
I wish I had this information before my tubal ligation…

It was your right to have been informed before hand of this information.
The issue of women not being informed is very serious.
This fraud and abuse is criminal. It is real and ongoing.

Only when laws are created that protect women will we begin to see change and begin to heal and resolve some of these issues.

We are committed to and working toward change: creating and putting in place laws that will protect a women's basic human rights of being informed of serious side effects and risks at the time of consent.

Only when a woman is fully informed will she be giving true consent.

"The better informed we are, the healthier we'll be!"

Coalition for Post Tubal Women - Mission Statement:

To educate, inform and provide accurate information to women considering tubal ligation. To educate, inform, assist, and create a supportive network for post tubal women in their quest for answers and proper follow-up care. To bring forth the needed change which would require women to be fully and properly informed prior to tubal ligation surgery.

Education Programs:

Education comes in many forms. This book, the tubal.org web site, outreach programs, and public lectures and workshops are just a few ways we are educating women about post tubal syndrome (PTS) and the issues at hand.

Change:
We are committed to and working toward "change". This involves creating and putting in place laws that will protect a woman's basic human rights of "being informed". Repeatedly we hear women stating, "I wish I had know this information before my TL". This issue of women not being informed is very serious. Only when laws are created that protect women will we begin to see "change" and begin to resolve some of these issues.

We are working within and networking with other organizations in order to accomplish these goals. The CPTwomen has gained the support of IL NOW (National Organization of Women) by their passing of the 1999 Tubal Ligation Resolution. We ask that all women join us and take a stand on this issue in order to create the needed change which will protect and benefit all women and our daughters that follow.

With proper laws in place doctors will be required to inform women of Post Tubal Ligation Syndrome. While our generation was not informed, working together we can break this cycle of abuse and ensure that future generations are informed.

Together we can make a difference!

Key issues are:

1. The ACOG publicly denies that tubal ligations cause such conditions as post tubal syndrome (PTS), bleeding disorders, or hormonal imbalances.

This issue can be directly compared to the tobacco companies withholding information from the public. The only difference is people who developed health problems from smoking they were not required to return directly the tobacco people for help and health treatment. When women develop PTS they have no choice but to return back to an obgyn doctor, and their organization (the ACOG) that withheld the information from them initially. Women are denied proper testing, diagnosis, and treatment. The code of silence is very strong.

2. Tubal ligations are known by the ACOG and their members to cause hormonal imbalances and other side effects. These side effects have been proven through clinical research and studies, and have been reported by health professionals and victims who have witnessed and experienced side effects first hand.

3. The Freedom of Information Act has allowed us to access studies proving. The ACOG is well aware of these studies, and writes and discusses these studies in their technical bulletins to their members. The ACOG in their bulletins directs their members to withhold the information, and the ACOG withholds this information in the patient information brochures that they provide to the public and to their members (obgyn doctors) to disperse among potential tubal ligation candidates.

The ACOG has conspired with malicious and wanton recklessness to keep this known information from the public for fear of the litigation that would ensue. They publicly refuse to acknowledge the scientific findings that prove such side effects are true and publicly state that tubal ligations do not cause such conditions. The ACOG and their members withhold this information from the public at large and no one is informed before or afterwards. Women are told afterwards that their current health condition could in no way have been caused by the tubal ligation surgery when there is no other cause. Post Tubal Women are denied testing, diagnosis, and treatment.

It is documented that after tubal ligation women are at higher rates for bleeding disorders, and hysterectomies. The ACOG and their members know that when tubal ligation surgeries are performed that many of the women will be returning for second and third surgeries such as D&C's and hysterectomies because of side effects from the TL, yet women are not informed of this risk at the time of consent.

The ACOG and their members withhold information and profit by doing so. They first profit when they perform the TL. They then go on to profit again from the original consumer fraud when performing second and third surgeries due to the result of the first surgery.

Women are not informed at the time of their TL that the surgery could create such conditions that would necessitate such treatments as D&Cs and hysterectomy. Women are told at the time of these second and third surgical producers that their tubal ligation surgery had in no way caused their health condition that necessitated such radical procedures.

Legal Issues include:
- Consumer Fraud
- Conspiracy
- Anti-Trust (RICO)
- Medical Tort/Battery
- Surgical Abuse
- Gross Negligence
- Violation of Civil Human Rights
- Discrimination
- And more

The CPTwomen has gotten much media attention with the "Campaign to Inform" and will continue to do so, as this is a women's health/consumer rights/human rights issue.

All post tubal women are asked to join the "Campaign to Inform" and take action.

No one is going to fight to create TL laws but us, we the women who have been victimized, injured, lied to and those who are angry and outraged that we were not informed.

It's not going to happen unless you and I make it happen.

No method is perfect, and all can cause PTLS - sjb

I'm mad as hell, cuz nobody, nobody told me!!!!!! - j

Letters and Statements to the CPTwomen

Introduction note: The following are copies of just some of the thousands of letters, statements, and postings that we receive on a day to day basis. I have duplicated the letters and statements just as they were received. I did not correct spelling errors and am not concerned with the spelling; it is the context of that's being said that is important.

    These letters and statements are presented so that women can see that they are not alone, and so the medical community can see what we, as women, are thinking and feeling as we leave their offices.

I had a tubal about 7 yrs ago and since that time i have exper an array of changes with my hormones, for one i will just go off at the drop of a dime for not reason half the time. I am tired most of the time and never felt the same since that surgery, My cycle has been much heavier. I was told by my doc that there were no bad side effects and that in fact i would exper better sex because the worry of pregnancy would not be there. I know several other people that have ha this surgery and have had adverse effects, much the same as i have had. I am now going through a health crisis that I think might be linked to the tubal. I am very tired still and very unable to concentrate, this has been going on for a while but it is only getting worse. I am only 32 and had my current doc tell me that i could be going through menapause, and that by having the tubal that this could make the symptoms of menapause arise sooner. Had i known that this would change my chemical make up I would have never had this sugery done. Instead i feel that i was lied to about the effects of it. I know now that this is such a huge part of us as women that it would only make sense that this would affect our bodies in some way, i just wish that i had known it then. Any info that you could send me on this would be very helpful,

thx Tammy

My wife was talked into tubal ligation by her OB/GYN without consenting me after our third child. I was under the impression that the Doctor viewed it, much like a car mechanic adding on other work, 'as long as he had the car up on the lift.'

At the particular time, I felt that my wife was in no condition, having just delivered our third child, to make a proper decision that was not based upon emotion.

We are not in dire financial straits, and I would love nothing more than to have another child.

I have noticed a dramatic change in her mood leading up to her periods. She will go from one EXTREME to another, often inciting arguments, destroying the sanctity of the home, only to have the waters calm dramatically after the menstration begins, to where I will be complimented on being a perfect, caring husband.

I would implore any woman considering such a venture to NOT entertain the idea within a year after having given birth.

Too often, the idea of a contraceptive procedure is far too alluring to a woman who has just given birth.

I feel that the AMA should address this type of predatory prospecting or the 'hawking of ovarian hacking,' because it preys on persons who may be in a compromised mental state. Particularly, women who have just given birth within the past year.

From a husband's perspective, it really takes it's toll upon, not only the marriage, but on the entire family as well. Not to mention the higher risk of coronary artery disease, and the acceleration of bone degenerative process--all this for a woman in the prime of her life. Sad, very sad. - John

---

Hello there - I just wanted to post this message to find out if anyone else has been diagnosed with ovarian cysts after having a tubal ligation. My 4th child was born in May, 2003, and I deciided to have a TL, thinking it was a sound, responsible decision. My husband would not even consider having a vasectomy, as I have come to find out, many don't! Anyways, the number of problems I have had to deal with is staggering, including heavy, painful periods, unbearable PMS, severe mood swings, hair loss, weight gain, especially around my waistline, I could go on and on. My doctor ordered a pelvic ultrasound two weeks ago, as I finally asked for help with my menstrual problems. The ultrasound came back abnormal, and the findings included multipe ovarian cysts and problems with the lining of my uterus. I am now scheduled for a biopsy next week with an OB/GYN that specializes in these types of issues. I cannot understand why so many of us were not treated with the dignity and respect we deserved, by not being told of the possible negative side effects of a TL. Thousands of smart moms out there cannot all be crazy!!! I hope to hear from some of you in this great forum that was set up for us. I am going to become a member of Tubal.org immediately. I hope you all hang in there, and that someday we will all see justice served to us. God bless you all - Sincerely, Amy

---

I am touched by all of your stories and will do my best to spread the word so that more women aren't blinded by this injustice. The sad thing is we as a society believe we can trust these doctors and that they are there to help us, to not only make the right choices for ourselves but to stay healthy in the process. It is unethical that this continues to go on. Women should be informed of this prior to signing on the dotted line. I want to do all I can to adovate for the women who have had this done as well as the women who haven't yet, to try to help prevent this from continuing on. I find it completely unacceptable that these doctors out there are not doing what is best for the woman in question, but what is best for their pocket book. To me this is just like medical malpractice. Doctors are supposed to take an oath to help people and their health, not hinder it as they do in this process. I am sincerely a new adovate of you all and this site. Thank You - Trish

---

Hi. I am new to this site and am so glad I found it. I just thought I was going crazy. I have three children and have seen two different doctors that have overlooked my problems. One doctor suggested I see a psychiatrist. The next doctor suggested I have a full historectomy & I am 27 years old. I am finally going to see a woman doctor on the 29th. I am not sure what can be done, I just want some relief from this rollercoaster life I have been living since my TL. - Living with PTLS - Deetra

---

I have been experiencing many of the symptoms of PTLS. Will tubal reversal help? - Tammy

---

I had a tubal 20 months ago because I was done having children, I have not been the same since, I am on anti depressants and one sleep aids to help me sleep at night, I am miserable. My kids are 3 and 19 months and sometimes I wish I didn't have them. I know it is terrible to say but they are driving me crazy. I know it is all to do with my post tubal syndrome. I do not know where to turn I had thought I had post partum depression but my baby is almost 20 mos old. What do I do now, I am at my wits end. Please help, should I get a reversal I would be willing to pay for it if it would help. - Alexandra

---

I had a tubal after my 4th child 2 1/2 years ago. When my periods returned they were like 4 times heavier than they had ever been in my life and they came every 2 or 3 weeks. I was scared I was hemoraging or something at first. My obgyn said it was just a normal change and to take ibuprofen to slow the bleeding. Now my hair has been falling out for over 6 months and I have facial hair that I guess isn't that bad, but it bothers me and it was never there before. I figured I must be starting menopause wicked early or something. I just turned 30 last month. I gain weight ten times faster than ever before and I just don't have my normal energy level anymore. I accidently came across something on the net that said post tubal litigation syndrome and it caught my interest. Now I am pretty upset considering I should have been told about this prior to the procedure. It all makes sense now, what's going on with my body, and it could have been prevented! I don't know how doctors can sleep at night. Not to mention it helps me none to know that a tubal reversal may help me, considering I have no insurance and am not wealthy. I should have researched it before I guess, but silly me I trusted my doctor to tell me of all the risks, not to pick and choose the ones that suited her needs. - Vikki

I think if a woman asks for a tubal ligation, she should be provided with information at the time she requests the tubal about how it can affect her physically and emotionally. For me, giving up my ability to have children, even though I technically don't want anymore, has had a HUGE mental effect on me. Women should have to review and sign this and return it to the doctor prior to the surgery. I know I signed consent for the surgery during admission to the hospital, but I signed a million papers then. I wasn't really taking all the tubal ramifications in during those few moments. - Anonymous

---

I'm now 26 years old a for the first time in my life I'm having painful cramps. Not to mention irregular periods and mood swings. Had I known all of the side effects possible from having a tubal ligation I would have made a different choice. That's the point "WE" should have been given all of the info to make an informed life altering choice! - Ginny

---

I descibe my symptoms, Mood swings, heavy bleeding, lasting 7-10 days, cramping before during and after my period, nausea and vommiting before and during my period, itchiness underskin (bad enough to scratch dinnerplate sized black bruises) non existant sex drive and pain during sex, headaches etc..

And they give me anti depressants saying it in my head....

Its not in my head these symptoms are very real....

I don't want to take anti depressants... I'm not depressed I am angry.

When i spoke of PTS the doctor spoke of PMS.

What can i do?... - Kathy

Wow! I am so gald I am not alone. I have went the last four years of my life being missed diagnosed. I had a tubal ringing in 1995. Subseqently, 10 years later I find myself to be overweight, fatigued, irritable, moody and want my life back. I am a registered nurse and would be glad to advocate to any OBGYN/MD that would listen to what we have to say. I have a lot of questions; Why wasn't this explained to us before the surgery, How can we reverse the situation, What research is actively be done, and What are the consequesces/leagal issues with doctors that have performed the procedure without fully understanding the outcome themselves. - Kim

---

I had a tubal ligation 2 1/2 yrs ago after the birth of my 3rd child at age 30. Since then I have experienced very heavy periods with a lot of clotting and cramping from ovulation to end of menstruation. 7 weeks ago I had a large cyst removed from my left ovary. The weekend prior to surgery I was very ill (period was extra heavy, vomiting, dizzy, pain in left shoulder blade) After surgery my OB said I was sick due to menstrual blood backing into my abdominal cavity---he was quick change the subject and simply prescribed the pill. I called the following week to ask if the bleeding was cyst related, he told me it was due to the ligation but would not go into detail---again quickly changing the subject and asking if I had my rx of pills to start first day of my next period and told me I was going to be just fine.

    I am very confused as to how this can happen, and very nerveous that it could happen again. I was hoping someone here could help explain this to me. Thank You, - Caryn

---

I went to my OB that did my tubal. She claimed the tubal was not the cause of all of these problems that i never had before (heavy periods, passing clots, cramping, migraines, nightsweats, hot flashes, no libido, no orgasm). She did bloodwork and found my estrogen in the post menopausal range (I was 30 at the time). Put me on the BCP then the patch, did a D&C to look for polyps (none were found).

After 3 years, I finally switched to a gyn with a good rep for hormonal knowledge. On the first visit, he told me he thinks its highly unlikely the tubal is causing my problems (here we go again!), but claims he'll be able to fix it. Just found a cyst on my left ovary, and wants me to have blood drawn at certain intervals of my cycle (never had that done before) to see what my levels are doing. We'll see I guess.....
- Allison

I went to my gyn although she was not the doctor that did the tl. She said the tl had no effect on the hormones, blood supply, etc. She did believe I had severe hormonal imbalance based on my symtoms, though (being more attributed to age, than the tl). She did a complete blood screen, tests for all hormone levels and a hormone saliva test. - Anonymous

update - My test results showed I have almost no progesterone-they are at levels of a menopausal woman. The doctor is relating this to my lack of menstruation due to breast feeding. Once I begin having a cycle we are going to test the levels again. - Anonymous

---

WHAT I WAS TOLD-

YES, THIS IS THE DOC. THAT DID MY T.L. THIS IS AT LEAST THE 4TH. TIME BACK COMPLAINING TO THE DOC. THE FIRST TIME I MENTIONED ANY OF THIS I WAS PUT ON ZOLOFT. OF COURSE THAT DID NOT CORRECT ANY OF THE PROBLEMS AND WAS OF COURSE TOLD IT WAS MY AGE OF WHICH AT THAT TIME WAS 29, AND THAT IT WAS MY AGE AND MY HORMONES AND NOT DUE IN ANYWAY TO YHE T.L. BACK AGAIN THEY DECIDED TO PUT ME ON EFFEXOR, AND EVEN SUGGESTED THE BIRTH CONTROL PILL TO CONTROL THE PERIODS IN WHICH I SAID NO. BACK FOR A RE-CHECK TO SEE HOW THE EFFEXOR IS DOING, IN WHICH THEY SUGGESTED A THYROID TEST AND FSH TEST AND ALSO DECIDED TO RAISE MY EFEXOR TO 150MG. FROM 75MG.

MY PHARMIST WAS GREAT AND REALLY TALKED TO ME ABOUT THIS, SHE SAID THIS IS SOMTHING SHE IS HEARING ALL THE TIME FROM WOMEN AND SUGGESTED I SHOULD GET MY HORMONES TESTED AND THEN SOME, AND TO REALLY READ THE SIDE EFFECTS OF THESE MEDICINES OUR DOCTORS OUR SO QIUCK TO PRESCRIBE. I FEEL LIKE A ZOMBIE WHILE ON THIS MEDICINE AND THEN SOME. AFTER GOING WHERE MY PHARMIST SUGGESTED

THEY SUGGESTED HRT, AND MY DOCTOR SAID IF THAT IS WHAT YOU WANT TO TRY, AND ALSO TOLD ME THE EFFEXOR SHOULD BE TAKING CARE OF ALL MY PROBLEMS, HOT FLASHES, NIGHT SWEATS ,MOOD SWINGS ETC.. ETC..

TAKE CARE ALL, - LISA

I had my tubal ligation done back on june 27th 2003. since then my periods went from 3 days to 8 days of constant heavy bleeding, I was never like this previous to my surgery. My mood swings are horrible for about 2 weeks prior to my period I go from sad to mad it is just crazy of course I told my doctor he said this is all because of my age and had nothing to do with my tubal, heck I just turned 31. I wake up in the night soaking wet , I have hot flashes all the time. The crazy thing is my friend told me not to do it because my recovery would be so much harder, so of course me and my husband asked the doctor about all of this and he basically made it sound like a walk in the park, he said we will be in there doing the c-section so why not! then I don't have to go through another surgery. well obviously he convinced us and here I am just wishing I could have my life back the way I was and felt prior to tubal ligation. - LISA

Boy, did my tubal ever go wrong...

Ironically, I had visited this site prior to my tubal, to get some stats on possible risks. I read with interest, but still decided the odds were in my favor. I did, however, ask my doc about post-tubal syndrome, and, although he was honest about it, he dismissed it as such a small risk, it wasn't worth considering.

I went in about 4 wks ago for day surgery...Sept. 8, 2004. It was only supposed to last 45 min. to an hour. After a really long time, the doctor burst into my recovery room, where they had told my husband to wait, and told my husband to start praying and contacting family...that I might not make it. My husband, in shock and weeping, started making calls to my and his families.

My doctor got in a hurry, I figure because he was running behind, and when he punched the trocar into me, he punctured my iliac artery. He, at least, knew he could in no way save me, himself, so he screamed for someone to get in there and help him. Two of the best surgeons in the hospital (one of them, a relative by marriage) responded, thank God, because they literally saved my life. They had to open me from my sternum down to my pelvic bone, to find the bleed. I had to have 13 units of blood replaced. I coded (vital signs ceased) at least once. The surgeons had to exert unbelievable pressure on the artery, while trying to tie off the artery. After the first surgery to stop the bleeding, the surgeon related to me by marriage spoke to the family. He told them I was stable, but he would have to immediately go back in for surgery. The pressure on my artery had caused a blood clot to form, and I had no circulation to my left leg. There was a real chance of amputation, right then.

He removed a large clot, and saved my leg. They moved me to ICU, and when I came to, I had a ventilator tube down my throat, my hands were tied to the bed rails, and my left calf muscle felt like it was literally about to explode. I couldn't talk, so I pointed to my leg, frantically, and made hand gestures to let them know there was something wrong with my leg. I couldn't even open my eyes, because the trauma of the surgery, and all the fluids they had pumped into me, caused my eyes to swell shut. My husband said I looked like "Rocky", the boxer, at the end of a match.

The surgeon did a doppler scan and found I had "compartmental syndrome" in my calf muscle, which is a result of the muscle trying to swell, after having lost blood flow, and the fascia, a tough membrane, preventing it from swelling. So, at 1 am, he had to take me BACK to surgery to save the leg again. He, later, told us that, when he cut the fascia, the muscle was under so much pressure that it sounded like a shotgun, when he made the cuts. My leg was saved, but I now have two teardrop shaped open wounds on either side of my calf, approx. 7 in. long and 3-4 in. wide. They have me on a wound vac, which is draining all the fluid and helping the leg to shrink enough so that they can take me back to surgery soon and sew the leg closed. Oh, and while he was in there, the surgeon decided to double check everything, and it's a good thing he did. He found and removed another large blood clot from my femoral artery in the top of my left leg, so I have yet another gnarly scar.

I am in constant pain, especially on the days the home health nurse comes to change my wound vac dressings (every other day). I am walking with a walker, and having to see physical therapists in my home to regain use of my leg. I am 34 years old, and I feel like an invalid. My life has been forever changed. I will never again refer to any surgery as "routine". And, now, I worry about long-term effects, such as post-tubal syndrome, etc. We have contacted an attorney and are taking this to litigation, for our family's sake. This is enough to destroy us, financially.

Has anyone else experienced such horrible an outcome from a "simple" procedure? - Angela

---

I ALMOST DIED FROM TL

I'll try to make a long stort short. Afetr having my third child at 30 yrs old I decided to have TL because my husband refused to have a

V. Well what was supposed to be an in & out surgery put my life in danger. I woke up after the surgery screaming in horrible pain, the nurses wouldn't listen to me and they told my mother that some women handle it better than others. Which my mother knew was BS becasue she knows how strong I am. Anyways, after awaking three times screaming and telling them I know something is horribly wrong with me please help me. And all three times they blew me off and gave me another shot to put me back to sleep. When my husband came in the Recovery Room I told him I think I'm dying something is very wrong! He then demanded that the nurses call my Dr. She ordered them to get an X-Ray and low & behold I was bleeding internally from a slice in one of my vessels. My belly was full of blood which is what put me in such pain. So I was rushed in for emergency surgery to repair the damage and I ended up having to stay in the hospital overnight.

After I got home I had major pains shooting down my legs and now I have horrible menstrual cycles with major cramps, bleeding & pain for like 10 days and the same pain in my legs. I also suffer from major pain on my left side all the time and the Dr. did many test and ultrasound to find that the scar tissue build up is the cause of my constant side pain which is even worse during intercourse. They told me there is nothing they can do for me and that I will just have to live with it.

This has ruined my marriage of 13 yrs because I do not want to have sex ever! So, anyone who is thinking about having this surgery SHOULD NOT!!! They do not tell you about these other crazy post surgery systoms. - TLC

Ovabloc

I am a 1981 clinical trial Ovabloc recipient who has been diagnosed with Multiple Sclerosis. I desperately need information about the silicone material used in this procedure. I fear that there may be many ill women out there. FDA will not help me and stated that they can only release the information to the corporation that paid for the clinical trial. I'm still shocked. One would assume that if FDA were overseeing a clinical trial, there would be some level of protection available for the participants. Thanks for your time.- Judy

---

tubes tied 12 years ago without knowing it!

As I was just diagnosed with andenomyosis and looking at surgery in less than a month, i thought i would do some research and came across this site. I had my daughter by c-section 12 years ago. While the doctor had me under, she walked out and asked my husband if they should tie my tubes. He said yes and that was that. When i mentioned days later I would like more children that is when my husband informed me I could not. Now I find out my current "problem" could have been caused by their action years ago! I am even more angry. - Julie

Hydrosalpinx 2 years after Tubal Ligation

  2 years ago I had a tubal ligation done. Never when discussing the risks was it revealed to me that I might need surgury again to correct complications from the first one! Last week I went to the ER with lower right pelvic pain thinking it was appendicitis. The appendicitis was ruled out pretty quickly but after an ultra sound and a CT scan, it revealed a scarey looking cystic like structure that was separate from the uterus and separate from the ovary. Immediately my husband and I thought the worst. When I followed up with my ob/gyn, he stated the he thought it was on my fallopian tube and that it was a hydrosalpinx that had become twisted. Apparently this is a pretty uncommon complication that can happen, but none the less a complication that should be discussed with people as a risk. Now I have to go back and have more surgery to remove the tube and possibly the ovary as well. Has any one else had this experience? I can't find much on this on the web either. – Jane

---

A hydrosalpinx occurs when a damaged fallopian tube fills with fluid.

A hydrosalpinx can occur anytime something happens to cause a fallopian tube to close. Fallopian tubes can close by injury or infection occurring to the end of the fallopian tube, the ampulla, and its delicate fingers, the fimbria, and by surgical means such as tubal ligation surgery. Glands within the tube produce a watery fluid that collects within the tube, producing a sausage shaped swelling that is characteristic of hydrosalpinx.

Thank you soooo much for this site. I literally thought that I was going crazy. Weird periods, forgetful, can't sleep, tired, moody, you name it. Sex drive, gone, zip. I had a tubal 4 years ago and my health has changed a lot! After being checked for a heart murmur I was given anti depressants and told that I was under stress and that it was all in my head. Now it all makes sense. - Liz

---

Doctor said ligation would not cause such things to happen

  I am 28 years old. I had a tubal ligation one year ago. Since then I have had these symtoms: No sex drive ,dry vagina, stomach aches, headaches, heavy periods, loss of short term memory ,crying all the time, mood swings ect. I have talked to my ob and he said the ligation would not cause such things to happen. I asked it he'd check my hormone levels and he refuses to order the tests.

  Please help me. - Jenna

I want to get involved

    I want to know how I can help getting women informend on this issue. This is something that is never talked about in the media. Yet other side effect of meds and procedures are. I guess you have to start in your own home town. Let me know what I can do. - Susan S

Heart troubles....

    I was wondering if there could be complications elsewhere besides ovaries and hormones..etc..

    I have developed heart palpitations and am currently looking for a cause..I don't drink/eat caffine products... and that is the main thing i know of that causes them... any information would be greatly appreciated...thanks! - tonia

(reply) Yes- read on.... by susan j bucher

    I am not a doctor, but this is what I understand to be true...

First of all if you are having palpitations this could be very serious. If you are anemic or suffering a hormone imbalance, which both could be caused from the tubal, you could experience palpitations. Known and common symptoms of anemia (low iron) include shortness of breath and heart palpitations, as well as the common "always tired"

    As far as hormones are concerned....The following are some quotes for a recent study (1997) about heart palpitations and women...

    Palpitations occur frequently in women at all ages, especially during the luteal phase (which is a hormonal phase) of the menstrual cycle... (tubal ligations can cause hormonal imbalances and create shorter, more intense luteal phases)

    A correlation between "ovarian hormones" and occurrence of paroxysmal supraventricular tachycardia (abnormal heart rhythms) has recently been reported in female patients with normal menstrual cycles; (meaning you may be still having regualr or semi regular periods, but the ovarian hormones, or lack of them could cause palpitations....)

    Palpitations during the perimenopausal period are usually benign and seem to be related to the increased sympathetic activity caused by the menopause (meaning palpitations during meno are common)

Again, I'm not a doctor, but if your experiencing palpitations due to lack of your "ovarian hormones" meaning "estrogen" you are probably experiencing bone loss as well.

Doc DENIED DENIED DENIED.

    I had my aptmt today.. the first words out of his mouth was. "Have we met, do I know you", I gave him a look like he was on drugs.. I said of course.. even my husband spoke up.. Stupid question.

    He told me that PTS does not exist that back in the 70's it was thought it was caused by TL but that it was dropped and has not heard of anything since then and that I am the first women to call this to his attention.

    Told him all the symptoms that I have been having and he said there is not proof that TL did this and that he is a scientific man and with out "black and white" evidence he can not help me. He then said that no one in the entire clinic would ever diagnose me with PTS as it doesn't exist. I can completely see the true code of silence at work here.. I am on my way to the clinic to get my medical records and then make copies of every thing and then give it back.. he said something very particular.. he said i will order the blood work. .but I can tell you now it will not help you.. it really will not help you, not that I am going to alter them or anything, you know because I have been here for 17 years and I can tell you they are not going to help.. WHY DID HE NEED TO SAY>>> not going to alter them or anything????? My husband did not even catch that. I just looked right at my husband with my eyes wide open. I want to get my records and have them copied so that at least for now I know that they are how they should be.. - Deborah

---

Former OB/GYN Office Nurse

    Hello, My name is Dana and I spent one and a half years working for an OB/GYN in his office. Before this, I was a Labor & Delivery nurse. I am now pregnant with my third son and have been thinking about having a BTL.

    I remember from working in the doctor's office, however, that many of our patients not only regretted the procedure some years later, but that many experienced the so called "complications": heavy menses, pain, and almost always ended up having to take birth control pills. I don't recall any developing adhesions but I didn't work there that long.

    I am glad to have found this site. I now know that it wasn't all in my head. I will not be getting a tubal. I feel good that at least on an individual basis while I was still working I did advise the patients on what I had "noticed" and advised them to talk about it with the doctor. - Dana

---

Dammed if they do or don't....

    I can understand physicians who actually do the surgery not wanting to acknowledge this, but what about the physicians that we all *are seeing AFTER the fact. My big question is WHY? What are THEY afraid of??? - Anomynous*

To answer your question regarding oaths...

Standard of Care: The uniform standard of behavior upon which the theory of negligence is based. - The standard of care requires the (doctor) to do what the "reasonable person of ordinary prudence" would do in the (doctors) place. If the (doctors) conduct falls below the standard that a reasonable person would conform to under like circumstances, the (doctor) may be liable for injuries or damages resulting from his or her conduct. (Copied from Blacks Law Dictionary.)

Physicians and attorneys are held to a higher standard of care than the lay person. They answer to a board of peers who usually judge their behaviors as doctors. Yes, I do believe they have a code of ethics. This is simialar to an attorney answering to a Law Board. Don't quote me, This is just what I "remember" from school. I havn't researched this part fully yet.

Consider this, If doctors are held to the same standard of care as their peers, Need I say more???? If their peers insist that PTS dosn't exist, where does that leave us????

Also, I'm wondering if the some physicians out there, are being held back by "managed care". I know that my physician has made mention to me that he no longer has the freedom to practice to his full ability due to the changes with managed care and hmo's. In the past two years I have seen him go from being a wonderful attentive person who researched EVERYTHING; to a doctor who is a slave to the insurance companies, and to the managed care facility that he works for. They refuse to allow him to limit his patient load. Instead of me getting a 1/2 hour to discuss my concerns with him, I have 15 minutes. That is NOT enough time to convince him of the changes that my body is going thru. It's barely enough to explain ONE symptom! So I keep going, until he is so sick of me, he'll have to do something. This tecnique of mine is paying off, luckily.

HOWEVER; I'm NOT saying that this is indicative to EVERY physician out there, but this could be a factor. Not everything is black and white. Some of the story's that I read posted here make me cringe. I cannot believe the doctors out there who refuse and disregard our rights.

Every situation is very unique, and needs to be delt with differently. I would never dream of suing my current physician. I understand his dilemma.

Sue the doctor who did my surgery??? You bet ya!!! Sue these bastards that call us crazy??? Sue the ones who blatantly DENY us testing?? You bet your ass we should sue. Or yell and scream until we get our way!

Doctors golden rule regarding the treatment of post tubal women.

1. Never hormone test post-tubal women. Avoid doing so at all costs.

2. put them on the pill, and no other forms of hormone treatment. Even if she is going into ovarian failure she'll never know because the pill will cause her to have monthly withdrawal bleeds. so what if the high amounts of estrogen can cause her to stroke out.

3. if her periods are heavy and she's in pain, offer a hysterectomy. If she doesn't opt for it right away, after being on the pill long enough she will, it's just a matter of time.

4. Tell her it's in their head and put her on antidepressants. So what if she has a hormonal imbalance that is causing a dementia type state. So what if she's having bone loss because she's suffering a progesterone/estrogen deficiency.

5. If a patient does request hormone testing, tell her they are very expensive (lie), that insurance won't pay for it (lie), that it won't show or diagnose anything (lie), that they are too young to be menopausal (lie), stall by saying that you have to research what tests to order, then say o.k., then order just a thyriod test and iron levels, but not the tests that would show her that she has a hormonal imbalance... when the tests come back tell her everything is fine.

- sjb

"Stress" the cause of the changes in your periods?

It's an insult to be told that "stress" causes changes in our periods....

It's "propaganda" and we are being told that it's in our "head".

Stress does not cause changes in our periods.

Hormones level changes, and other conditions can, but stress..... no.

Can a hormonal level imbalance cause us to be under stress? yes, but the "stress" is caused by the results of the imbalance which is caused by the TL.

Can "stress" alone cause changes in our hormonal balance??? no.

This has never been proved. - SJB

I went to the new doc yesterday. He spent over 2 hrs. with me and listened to everything I had to say. He did say that PTS does exist he felt that it is rare.(?) After what I have seen here it can't be all that rare. He did say that he would be willing to work with me but he wants to get ALL my records from my previous doc. He was concerned about all the things I have gone through and he said the doc that I had been seeing was to willing to due surgerys. (He wanted the big bucks) He has not ordered any test yet he said he wanted to go over the previous reports then make a clean start. He is going to make copies of those reports for me. He even question the anti-depressant I was given after being in the hopital for 4 days with an infection that I believe was caused by the doc (being that one hand was in a cast while performing a hystascope proceedure in his office). I don't know but I think this is a good start. I just feel so let down by the other doc and so angry.I want these problems fixed NOW but I know this is going to take some time. - Robin

---

You can use this in the book- I flew to German to give my paper on the need for proper informed consent for BTL.

    The French MD's felt that he need was there to change and talked with me. My talk was covered by the German Press. I had released data showing how many women were having severe problems after BTL. The USA md's hated my talk and attacked me on the floor during the Q and A session. I was well prepared and made them look more and more stupid as they asked questions and began to show they had knowledge and were not treating these women. In the end I exposed all that I wanted to and more. By attacking me I was able to open up their own compliance.

    The woman interviewed me for an hour. The piece never ran. When I was done the German and USA heads went to her and told her if she printed the paper it would cause havoc and women would sue their MDs.

    She said no she was going to print it . The GYNS then had 20 MD's call her threatening to sue the paper. It was never printed.

This was 1991....

My paper was peer reviewed and all the data was proven .... - VGH

---

dogma

dogma n 1: a religious doctrine that is proclaimed as true without proof [syn: belief, tenet] 2: a doctrine or code of beliefs accepted as authoritative

---

DOG MA MA

1/ BTL has no side affects

2/ Your complications after a BTL are all in your head

3/ A hysterectomy will cure you

4/ Trust me

5/ Reversal will solve your problems

ALL ARE DOG MA MA - Dr. VGH

This is not a year I have any caring for men
I am bitter and do not like men in general
and seeing how they stick together against women.. so that is my head
However ..there is data to show many many complications from Vas..
1/anti sperm antibody formation
2/pain and infection
3/increase CAHD

these papers exist and have been covered up - VGH

Medical Dogma

These are key words or phrases that need to be used consistantly, in order to help shear the semantical alpaca from the ears of the customers of the male medical monopoly : Castration(res ipsa loquator), Prevailing incorrect opinion of the male medical majority, medical monopoly, cookbook medicine, Simon Says medical education, Medical lobbist in congress, paternalism, uninformed consent, doctor/customer power exchange, ritual mutilation, medical dogma, respect of customer intelligence, medical library, medical history, research and customer autonomy reigns supreme. - walker

---

PAIN ISSUE - VGH

PAIN - This is to be placed on the web under education.

1/Document your pain - Make a monthly calander and document our pain

2/Get the operative report of your BTL

3/Get the pathology report of your BTL

4/Get any photos of your BTL

5/Have a full hormonal evaluation

6/Have a full evaulation for STD

7/Have a pelvic ultrasound

8/Report your complication here on this web site

9/If a device was used (Hulka Clip, Fallop Rings, Fishie Clip, etc Report this to the FDA in a formal device form

These are the first steps. This is educational material only.

I have read so many of these messages and see myself in all of them. I had my tubes tied the day after my son was born in 1996. I was not told anything about the side effects. Problems soon started (too many to list). I tried BC Pills and hormones and after 10 months of bleeding 15-18 days a month and almost constant PMS I was advised to have a hysterectomy. It was going to cure all of my problems. The doctors don't tell you anymore than they do for the Tubal. I now have some other Menopause problems that I knew nothing about and feel that I made 2 BAD CHOICES. I have found a Hysterectomy Support Site and have told my story so that maybe things like this won't happen anymore. By the way I'm 32 and 7 mos. Post hysterectomy and on more meds and vitamins to try and fix things than you can shake a stick at!! - Julie

---

Had Exploritory Surgery....

I have a question....I had a Lap done two days ago. The doctor told me she found that the vein going to my right ovary is enlarged to 3 times its normal size??? She said that the blood has backed up in that vein and enlarged it. What does that mean....Is the supply of blood to that ovary diminished??? She also said I have Ademo (not sure how that is spelled) and the only answer is hysterectomy.

I was in recovery when she told me this ha ha ha...was to drugged up to ask her anything. - by Trish

---

Are there differences in the incidence of Post Tubal Ligation syndrome related to the way the sterilization was done? For example: unipolar and bipolar coagulation, falope rings, Hulka and Filshie clips, Pomeroy method. I'm curious which type of tubal blocking gives the best and worst results.

All the methods can cause PTS, but we believe the highest rate is when the tube is burnt.

This method (cauterization) happens to be the most popular way for doctors to perform the surgery. Almost all tubals are done this way.

Bands and clips can also cause the blood supply to be affected, but they are more easily reversed. Because bands and clips are made from metal (clips) and plastic's (clips and bands), women can develop allergic reactions to them, such as the breast women developed with the silicone breast implants, etc. The clips have been known to lodge into other organs, ect...

No method is perfect, and all can cause PTS. - Coalition Post Tubal Women

I wish I would of found this site 2 yr ago

Thank goodness! I finally feel like I have found some answers to all of my questions! Two years ago, after the birth of my third child, I too had a tl and now I am regretting it. I thought because of my age (36)then, that I should go ahead and have the tl done. Plus my insurance was to run out the end of that month. Now I wish I would of seen this site and had the knowledge that I do now. I have had so many problems with my periods and pms, irritability, mood swings, and probably the worst according to my husband is the loss of libido. I now have the most horrible thoughts about sex, which was never a problem before. Before the tl we had a healthy normal sex life and now I could care less if I ever do it again. I have not been to a doc yet, I'm not sure what can be done to "fix" all that is broken since having the tubal. My only hope is that anyone who is thinking about having a tl done, please rethink it and get more info. I would not have done it if I had know what the after effects were. - Jen

---

WAS NEVER INFORMED

i had a t.l. 2 years ago at age 36. i had most of the symptoms listed almost immediately. i went back to the doctor that did the surgery,he said my symptoms had nothing to do with the surgery. it was post partum depression and would go away. well it didnt,in the mean time i went on the internet and found alot of information, things the doctor never mentioned to me. in fact i wasnt even given a brochure to read, i didnt know anything about having the gas put into my abdomen and i woke up with having more pain than i ever had giving birth my four children, which all weighed 10 pounds each. i wasnt told that it was going to be so painful. the only thing my doctor told me was that i now have very large adhesions internally which i can feel through my abdomen and he gave me anti-inflammatory prescription for. which didnt make the adhesions go away. i still have stinging pain from that. i went to another doctor,after reading this, i told him all my symptoms and didnt mention post tubal syndrome. he told me right away i had a hormaonal imbalance, and i should be tested. that was until he asked me about my birth control method and i told him i had a tubal then he quick changed his mind. and then i said the tubal has something to with it doesnt it, and he said ..people just like to think it does. he refused to order the hormone testing. he said your hormones shift so much anyway it wont tell me any thing. and all he really cared about was who did the surgery (i think they all like to stick up for one another) and he said i want you to take the birth control pills. and if you want i can prescribe prozak for the depression and mood swings. i said no .. forget it. in the meantime i was in a very severe state of depression, crying all the time. i couldnt hardly take care of my baby and my 3 year old, or my two teenagers. my husband was of no help, he didn't want to read any of the information on the internet. or anything that i had to say about it. during this time we were divorced because of this.

i later found a female doctor who immmediately told me that it was post tubal syndrome, she did nothing about the depression. she did give me a low dose birth control pill, which mentally did make me feel better, my mind felt clearer, but i had to go through all the things that i never liked about being on the pill before. i was off the pill almost 10 years because i didnt like the side effects. i gained 17 pounds in the 2 months that i was on them so i went off of them. she told me that she would prescribe another b.c. pill if that one didn't work. i asked her about hormonal testing she didn't want to do that. she said it wasn't really necessary. my periods are irregular, and after my periods are over i have a bloody discharge for about a week. also while she was doing the examination, she told me that my uterus was enlarged, which she said probably fibroids, and as she presses on my right side it hurt really bad and i jumped when she did that. she said oh, i hit your ovary. I have never had that kind of pain during an exam, she didnt say why it would hurt like that. should i be concerned? my left one didnt hurt. since my surgery i have had the weight gain, up and down, major depression which feels like post partum depression that will never go away. uterine pain almost all the time. irregular periods, major mood swings.trouble sleeping, no libedo, dry irritated vagina,severe anxioty, fatigue, my skin itches, my muscles ache all the time, i am very active. i have hair loss and dizziness. i have become so forgetful. my friends say that i was so healthy looking before the surgery and i am so ill looking now. none of my friends will have this done after they have seen what i have been through. - tina

---

I have decided to talk my wife out of this procedure!!!

After reading all the horror stories of this procedure, I am horrorified. I love my wife with all my heart and soul and I can not let this happen to my wife. She is due soon(June 25, 2000). And we already signed the forms but, that will change come her next appointment. Thank so much for this info. I can never tell you all the diference in me, and I am a man. Once again, Thank You All - Mike

---

Mad as hell, cuz nobody, nobody told me!!!!!!

I had my tubal 3 years ago after the birth of my fourth child, I was 23 years old. When I first complained about the differences in my menstruel cycle, like ohhh gee I di'dnt have any real "cycle" to speak of any more; either my periods were ridiculously early as much as two weeks early or very late, as much as 4-6 weeks late, I was told by my doctor whom I trusted that it was only my body adjusting to the birth of my last child and had nothing to do with my tubal

OK- what ever. A part of me still believed him then even though I strongly suspected it was the tubal since with all 3 of my other children my body had "adjusted" with in 6 months. This was about 1 year after my tubal.

Well here I am and my periods are still screwed up, to add to that now my PMS is twice as worse as it ever was before, in the past I had fairly mild PMS, these days I have been sooo moody I've even had suicidal thoughts, my back aches, my head aches, my breasts ache, when my period bothers to show up I'm in bed for the first 3 days with severe cramps, I get diareaha, my flow is much heavier enough that just using a tampon or pad (or both for that matter) is'nt enough protection. I've taken to using the "instead" cup which one is supposed to be able to wear twice as long as a tampon or pad however I find myself needing to change because it is full as often as every two hours.

My doctor has just prescribed the pill for me. I'm going to take it because I am so miserable but I'm mad as hell about all of this. He still denies that it has anything to do with my tubal he says it's my aging. MY AGING??? at 26 is it normal for a woman to be in perimenopaus??? If I wanted to take the pill I would'nt have had the tubal. If I had known this would have happend, I would'nt have had the tubal.

Last year a dear friend of mine had a tubal, she was 24. I begged her not to, I told her what happend to me. Her doctor told her that post tubal syndrome is something that women who regret their tubals because they want to have more children have. BULL. I'm very fulfilled with my four children and do not wish to have more. Unfortunately my friend is now also experiencing nearly the same symptoms as myself. but it has nothing to do with the tubal the doctors say. bull. - by Janice

---

my doctors a fool

i went back to the doctor who gave me my tubal, for the 100th time, i asked him to check my hormone levels , he said he thinks its a good idea for me to have an exploratory surgery, i said not until you run some other tests ,I'm not looking forward to being cut open again, and I'm tired of this. I'm going to get another opinion, so i made an appt with another gyn. ..when i called the office the doctor got right on to ask me what was going on i told her my symptoms, and that it started after my tubal, she said it is possible my tubal caused these problems, i hope she can help me - theresa

---

ADHESIONS ON UTERUS

Well, I ended up in the emergency room this morning. I went due to a upper respiratory infection I have had for the last two weeks, but when they asked me when my last period was and I told the nurse which one she looked surprised. I told the attending ER physician about the pain I have had for the last nine years on my left side. Well I got a catheter to fill my bladder and they did an ultrasound on me. The Dr. came to me about an hour later, and I guess he thought he was funny, he said" well, I have good news, you r not pregnant." But that I do have adhesions on my uterus, and that happens alot with women who have had tubals, and that all he could tell me was to have another surgery, but that may not help, it may make it worse. So, in not so many words he was telling me that I needed a hysterectomy, what other "surgery" would he be talking about? But at least now I have it documented that I have had an ultrasound, and a witness to what he told me, my sister in law was there with me through it all. So, anyone else out there been through this part of it, and just what are adhesions? - Nicole

I am so happy that I found this website...

I had my tubal in Feb. of 96. I would say that within 6 months of having it done I started to have female problems. My periods became real irregular. Some months I would flood while others a day or two of what I would call on again and off again spotting. I began to have numerous bladder infections. I started to have heavy pre menstral cramping, something that I had never experienced before. When I would ovulate I would always know it, because the pain on either side was terrible. I started having alot of stomach problems such as ulcers and acid reflux. I got numerous gallstones which resulted in having my gallbladder removed in 97. I have night sweats, hot flashes, weight gain, nauseated all of the time, I am tired all of the time. Sex is VERY painful. I get shooting pains that start in the center of my lower abdomen, and radiate all the way through my anus.

All of these things I see are symptoms of PTLS. I can tell you this my gyn. never ever informed me of these side effects. The only things that he said is there was a 1 and 40,000 chance of me becoming pregnant and that If I did get pregnant my chances of a tubal pregnancy were like 1o times more likely. He never said that my life would be a living hell, and that I would experience menopausal symptoms at 25 yrs. age. I am 29 now.

I hope that there is a class action lawsuit. I want to be right there in that action to when It is filed, because If I would have known about all of these numerous health problems that getting my tubes tied would cause I think that I would have toughed it out and lived off of the depo shot or the pill.

Again I am so happy that I found a place to talk to women that are just like me. Women that struggle with this pain each and every day. To be honest if I do have a laparoscopic procedure done I am frightened at the mess my tubes are probably in now. Lets all get together and show our Dr's that they need to inform of of these problems and not just worry about making another dollar. I want this to stop. I want our dr's to be more upfront with us. Just maybe if they did that there would be alot less women on message boards such as this. I hope to hear from some more of you, and lets stick together and get something done for the mutilation that has happened to our lively hood.
- Priscilla

My Complications

First of all, I'd like to say that this is the first time since I had my tubal ligation almost two years ago that I've done any research on it and I am apalled! I came accross this website almost on accident and I'm glad I did. I cannot believe that these doctors and hospitals are getting away with this.

In Dec. of 1999 I gave birth to a daughter. She was my fifth child and I didn't want anymore (and my mother insisted that I didn't have anymore) so without much hesitation, I told my physician that I wanted a tubal ligation. She really didn't discuss anything with me at all, just got the paper work together, I signed it and it was all set up.

I nursed my daughter, so the first 3 or 4 months after having her, I didn't have a period at all, and I didn't think anything of it. When I finally did have one, it was awful. It felt like someone was ripping my insides out and I was flowing so heavy that you would've thought the same. At first, I shrugged it off, thinking that it was because I hadn't had one. Then, the next month, the same thing hapend, the next month, it happend again. Finally, aboout 4 months after having irregular, heavy bleeding, I knew something wasn't right. I started counting the days in between. There were only between 16 and 21 days after I stopped that I started again, and it lasted for at least 6-7 days. Every month is worse than the last. Some days, I can't even get out of bed. My stomach aches all the way down to my feet. And more often than not, I have severe pelvic pain, even in between cycles.

Finally, I made an appointment with my Dr. I told him what had been happening. He told me he'd never heard of a woman's period being worse after a tubal!! He offered to put me on the pill to see if that would regulate me, but I didn't want to be on the pill (that sort of defeated the purpose of having my tubes tied). He said I could have endometriosis. I thought maybe I was crazy, but now I know I'm not!

I am now (after reading what's poster on this webpage and several others) going to find a new physician and see what can be done (if anything) to help me. I am also going to seek legal advice as I think that physicians and hospitals should be held accountable for their inconsiderate actions. Why are we not being informed of the risks?

We need to take a stand and do something about this problem. - Sara

---

I think I'm menopausal!

I want to say thank you for this site. I just came upon it a few days ago. I never heard of post tubal syndrome. I showed the information to my husband and he agrees that this fits me to the T. I had a tubal ligation 5 years ago during my last c-section. My life (and his) since then has nothing short of misery. For at least the past two years I've been having irregular cycles, I can't sleep, I'm tired, moody, forgetful, depressed, I have hot flashes, and I have NO SEX DRIVE. I'm only 33 years old but feel like I'm 63. - Barb

---

Finally.........some answers. Let me start by telling you that I am 28 years old, have 4 children ages 2, 5, 7 & 8, I had my TL on October 15, 1999, the day after my daughter was born.

For the past two years I have believed that I am going crazy. I have had hot flashes, chills, mood swings, crying bouts, what I thought were anxiety attacks, horribly painful periods (it feels like a knife going straight through my lower abdomon), heavy periods with huge clots that are lasting a week. In the past two years I have often joked with my husband about feeling like I was going through menopause (menopause at 26-28?) Last week I went to my family practice doc and told him about these symptoms and I told him that they started occuring after my TL and birth of my child. He diagnosed me with depression and panic disorder and put me on Prozac and Xanax. I decided to research the depression on the internet and came across a site about post tubal ligation syndrome. A light bulb went off instantly. This site listed all of the same symptoms that I am having. I posted on a tubil ligation site only to be bombarded by posters who do not believe that this syndrome is real. I know that it is although I do believe that it may not occur in all women. I am making an appointment to demand that my hormone levels be checked. Can hormone replacement therapy help? I'm 28 and refuse to live my life like this. I feel so cheated that I wasn't told of any of these side effects no matter how small the risk. I don't think that I would have had the surgery. Thanks for listening. - Carmen

---

THE STORIES I HAVE READ (and what) SUSAN WROTE IS MY STORY TO A T.

IT IS UNFORTUNATE THIS HAS HAPPENED AS I ALMOST LOST (DID) LOSE MY LIFE LITERALLY AND DEFINITELY IN A MANNER OF SPEAKING.

I ALSO THOUGHT I HAD ALZHEIMERS. WHATEVER IT WAS IT DIDN'T EXIST EXCEPT I HAD GONE THROUGH MENOPAUSE.

I'M HURT, ANGRY, SHOCKED, RELIEVED, AND READY FOR A FIGHT.

I KNEW WHAT A TL WAS AND WHAT I WAS DOING OR SO I THOUGHT. HAD I KNOWN MY OVARIES WOULD CEASE TO FUNCTION AFTERWARD I MIGHT HAVE THOUGHT DIFFERENTLY OR AT LEAST NOT BEEN PUT THIS HELL ON EARTH WE CALL LIFE.

THE DAY I HAD SURGERY MY 6TH SENSE PICKED UP ON SOMETHING THE DOCTOR SAID RIGHT BEFORE I WENT UNDER.

I ALSO HAD VERY REGULAR PERIODS UNTIL TL. HE ASSURED ME I WOULD NEVER HAVE ANOTHER CHILD AS HE WOULD MAKE SURE OF IT. AT THE TIME I SHUDDERED AND THOUGHT THAT STATEMENT WAS INAPPROPRIATE. I DIDN'T GET A VERY GOOD FEELING FROM THAT STATEMENT AND ASKED MYSELF "WHAT IS HE GOING TO DO, MUTILATE ME?"

I THINK SOME DOCTORS ARE DOING THIS TO MAKE SURE WOMEN DON'T COME BACK WITH AN ACCIDENTAL PREGNANCY.

THIS IS HORRIBLE!!!!!!!!!! IT IS A CRIME.

AFTER SURGERY I NEVER HAD ANY MORE PERIODS. I WAS 37.

I WAS TESTED BY MY FAMILY DOCTOR AND MY TEST RESULTS WERE CONSISTENT WITH FEMALE MENOPAUSE. I WONDERED IF THIS WAS A SIDE EFFECT OF THE SURGERY AND AT THE TIME I SHRUGGED IT OFF AS MY IMAGINATION LIKE EVERYTHERE ELSE. I WAS TOLD THAT WAS OK. DON'T WORRY ABOUT IT. I WAS 38 NOT 57. - ROBIN.

Actions to Take

Today I work at a doctor's office. I love my job. It's low stress compared to other jobs I have had. Everyone is nice and I like seeing how everyone interacts. I do not talk about my tubal, that I have had a tubal ligation, or that I have done health rights activist work in the past. I don't talk about the tubal issue to these people because first of all this isn't the forum to do so, and second of all I'm burnt out. I know that talking to the people I work with is not going to make any real changes in the world.

In speaking out publicly about the in justices of women's health care regarding tubal ligation and informed consent, some people view me as a radical feminist. I do not feel like a radical feminist. I'm a regular mom with two kids living in suburbia going to soccer games and the grocery store. I had a tubal ligation for the purpose of birth control at the suggestion of my doctor. The doctor failed to warn me that tubal ligations had negative side effects, and when I returned to him in failing health he failed to help me. I am just a woman who wants the medical community to change the way they inform women about the risks of the surgery.

I wasn't informed before the surgery of the risks and the Ob/Gyn community is O.K. with that. I'm not O.K. with that. It's not right. Losing my ovarian function affected me physically and psychologically. I was not warned that this could occur. No one is warned, and the Ob/Gyn community is O.K. with that.

There's an old saying, "the squeaky wheel gets the oil." The medical community is not going to change on their own. The only way anything is going to change is if enough people make their voices heard.

There's another saying, "The nail that sticks out gets hit on the head". Singularly, that's what occurs, but if enough of us stick out, the system will have to be repaired.

The CPTwomen often receives letters asking, "What can I do to help?"

Your first and foremost action any woman should take is that of maintaining or improving your health. With out good health you can not work to make other changes. Your first action should be addressing your health. Get your hormones tested, and physical and mental health in order.

Sometimes becoming an activist and working to make social changes can help emotional health and healing. This is the route that I choose and hope that you can too.

The Campaign to Inform

In 1999, when I presented NOWs Tubal Ligation Resolution one woman stated to me that this issue was following in the footsteps of the Silicone Breast Implant Issue. NOW was very instrumental in their fight against the makers of the implants and laws surrounding their use. Still, they needed to be educated and informed of what the issue was and how it negatively affected women and women's rights. The Coalitions "Campaign to Inform" is just that, informing everyone of the issues at hand.

The CPTwomen aim is to put in place an informed consent law for tubal ligation. In order to do this the public must be informed not only of the complex issues at hand such as what post tubal ligation syndrome is, but also why there is a vital need for an informed consent law. The Coalition for Post Tubal Women's "Campaign to Inform" is targeted at all sectors of the public, from the lay person to doctors and lawyers.

To inform the public women are asked to speak up. Talk to your friends. Who else do you know who had a tubal with a change of health afterwards? Who else would be willing to help you write some letters or gather some petition signatures?

Write letters and contact your State Representatives and the Media. Women and the public need to be educated about the issues and informed. Your State Rep needs to be informed that you were not. It is advocated that you write to three of each.

Our State Reps have to see that we are serious about this being done. Provide them with a copy of this book, along with letters or petitions asking that they endorse a law.

Call or write a letter to your local news paper. Tell them what happened, or is happening to you and your friends health wise. Provide them with a copy of this book. When you call or write to your local media, tell them that you've collected petitions aimed at your state rep to take action.

While we were not informed, we can work toward ensuring that other women in the future are. You can take pride in knowing that you are working to make changes that will benefit women for generations to come.

Take Action!

- Join the National Organization for Women and attend meetings.
- Write and send letters to three of your State Representatives and ask that they endorse and support a "Tubal Ligation Informed Consent Law."
- Contact three of your local media (TV news, newspapers, radio) and ask them to report about the risks of tubal ligation and about the "debated" issues of non-consent and the need for a law.
- File your personal complaints of having not been informed to your State Medical Board.

The National Organization for Women (NOW)

NOW stands for the National Organization for Women. NOW's goal since its beginning has been to bring about equality for women.

NOW's official priorities are pressing for an amendment to the U.S. Constitution that will guarantee equal rights for women; achieving economic equality for women; championing abortion rights, reproductive freedom and other women's health issues; supporting civil rights for all and opposing racism; opposing bigotry against lesbians and gays; and ending violence against women.

NOW works on a wide variety of issues, including lobbing to make contraception (the pill) available to women who have a prescription (some pharmacist refuse to fill these orders because of their personal beliefs), lobbing to have insurance companies pay for the pill (many insurance companies cover prescription drugs but not the pill), as well as other women's health rights issues such as the silicon breast implant issues.

The issue of women not being informed of the risks of tubal ligation and the need for a law that requires doctors to inform women is a NOW issue and has already gained NOW's support with the passing of the 1999 Tubal Ligation Resolution.

If you really want to help and really want to see a change occur I suggest that you join your local NOW group or in the very least attend a meeting and ask for a few minutes to speak. NOW is the proper forum to speak out about this issue. Explain who you are, why you are there (to educate them about this non-consent issue), and what your goals are (to see that an informed consent law be put in place). The more women who join NOW or address NOW to educate them and speak out about this issue, the quicker we will see the change occur.

State and Local Medical Boards

Each state has a governmental regulatory board that serves to protect citizens form unethical doctors or dangerous medical practices. Their duties include licensing doctors, overseeing the activities of the physicians who offer services in their state, investigating when a complaint is made, and disciplining doctors when their actions merit so. Disciplinary actions can range from ordering further education and training to revoking the physicians medical license.

As a consumer of medical services you have a right and a duty to wage a complaint if you believe you were uninformed, mislead, treated unfairly, or injured by a physician or while in any medical setting. If your physician did not properly inform you before your tubal ligation, if your current doctor is not offering you help or treatment, or if any doctor or medical professional in any field of practice has ever acted unethically or inappropriately, your state board needs to be notified.

This is very easy to do.

The first step is to write a brief outline of what occurred (ie, Doctor failed to inform me). Locate your state medical board and submit your complaint. At the end of this section is a list of all the medical boards in the US.

State Medical Regulatory boards require that you complete an official form when submitting a complaint to them. Some boards have websites which offer electronic complaint filing or forms that can be printed, completed, and sent. If they do not have on-line forms, call them and ask that they send you a form.

After your State Board receives your complaint, they will contact you to confirm your complaint and to begin their inquiry into your reported matter.

Filing a complaint with your state medical board is not a lawsuit. Filing a complaint with your state medical board does not mean they will act to discipline the doctor or that they will even investigate your complaint. Many cases are "closed" without ever being "opened". The system is not perfect. In my case I found it to be laden with corruption. Still, it's the system that we are given to work with and it needs to be utilized. Your action may aid another women from the same treatment that you occurred. As State medical boards receive more and more complaints of the same manner, they will eventually be required to act.

See below to find your state medical board:

US State Medical Boards

Alabama State Medical Board
848 Washington Street, Montgomery, AL 36104
(334) 242-4116 (334) 242-4155 (fax)

Alaska State Medical Board
333 Willoughby Avenue, 9th Floor, Juneau, AK 99801
P.O. Box 110806, Juneau, AK 99811
(907)-465-2541 (907) 465-2974 fax

Arizona Board of Medical Examiners
1651 E. Morten Avenue, Suite 210, Phoenix, AZ 85020
(602) 255-3751 (602) 255-1848 (fax)
www.state.az.us/licensing.html

Arkansas State Medical Board
2100 Riverfront Drive, Suite 200, Little Rock, AR 72202
(501) 296-1802 (501) 296-1805

Medical Board of California
1426 Howe Avenue, Suite 54, Sacramento, CA 95825
(916) 263-2382 (916) 263-2487 (fax)
www.medbd.ca.gov/

Colorado Board of Medical Examiners
1560 Broadway, Suite 1300, Denver, CO 80202-5140
(303) 894-7690 (303) 894-7692 (fax)
www.dora.state.co.us/medical/

Connecticut Department of Public Health - Physician Licensure
410 Capitol Avenue, Initial MS#12APP, Hartford, CT 06134-0308
(860) 509-7563   (860) 509-8457 (fax)

Delaware Board of Medical Practice
Cannon Building, Suite 203, P.O. Box 1401, Dover, DE 19903
(302) 739-4522   (302) 739-2711 (fax)

District of Columbia Board of Medicine
614 H Street, N.W., Room 108, Washington, DC 20001
(202) 727-5365   (202) 727-4087 (fax)

Florida Board of Medicine
2020 Capital Circle S.E., Bin C03, Tallahassee, FL 32399-3253
(850) 488-0595   (850) 922-3040 (fax)
www.doh.state.fl.us

Composite State Board of Medical Examiners of Georgia
166 Pryor Street, S.W., Atlanta, GA 30303-3465
(404) 656-3913   (404) 656-9723 (fax)
www.sos.state.ga.us/ebd-medical/

Hawaii Board of Medical Examiners
1010 Richard Street, Honolulu, HI
96801, P.O. Box 96813, Honolulu, HI 96813
(808) 586-2708

Idaho State Board of Medicine
280 N. 8th Street, Suite 202, State House Mall, Boise, ID 83720
P.O. Box 83720, Boise, ID 83720-0058
(208) 334-2822   (208) 334-2801 (fax)

Illinois Department of Professional Regulation
320 W. Washington Street, 3rd Floor, Springfield, IL 62786
(217) 782-8556   (217) 782-7645 (fax)
They also have a Chicago Location -
www.state.il.us/dpr

Indiana Health Professions Board
402 W. Washington Street, Room 041, Indianapolis, IN 46204
(317) 232-2960   (317) 233-4236
www.ai.org/hpb

Iowa State Board of Medical Examiners
1209 E. Court Avenue, Executive Hills West, Des Moines, IA 50319
(515) 281-5171   (515) 242-5908 (fax)
www.docboard.org   e-mail: ibom@adph.state.ia.us

Kansas State Board of Healing Arts
235 South Topeka Boulevard, Topeka, KS 66603-3449
(785) 296-7413   (785) 296-0852 (fax)
www.ink.org/public/boha

Kentucky State Board of Medical Licensure
Hurstbourne Office Park
310 Whittington Parkway, Suite 1-B, Louisville, KY 40222
(502) 429-8046   (502) 429-9923 (fax)

Louisiana State Board of Medical Examiners
630 Camp Street, New Orleans, LA 70130
P.O. Box 30250, New Orleans, LA 70190-0250
(504) 524-6763   (504) 568-8893 (fax)

Maine Board of Licensure in Medicine
137 State House Station, Augusta, ME 04333
(207) 287-3601   (207) 287-6590 (fax)
www.docboard.org

Maryland Board of Physician Quality Assurance
4201 Patterson Avenue, P.O. Box 2571, Baltimore, MD 21215-0002
(410) 764-4777   (410) 352-2252 (fax)
www.docboard.org

Massachusetts Board of Registration in Medicine
10 West Street, Boston, MA 02111
(617) 727-3086   (617) 451-9568 (fax)
www.docboard.org

Michigan Dept. of Consumer & Industry Services
611 West Ottawa, First Floor, Lansing, MI 48933
P.O. Box 30670, Lansing, MI 48909
(517) 335-0918   (517) 373-2179 (fax)
www.cis.state.mi.us/ohs

Minnesota Board of Medical Practice
2829 University Avenue, S.E., Suite 400, Minneapolis, MN 55414-3246
(612) 617-2130   (612) 617-2166 (fax)
www.bmp.state.mn.us

Mississippi State Board of Medical Licensure
2600 Insurance Center Drive, Suite 200-B, Jackson, MS 39216
(601) 354-6645   (601) 987-4159 (fax)
www.msbml.state.ms.us

Missouri Board of Registration for the Healing Arts
3605 Missouri Boulevard, Jefferson City, MO 65109
P.O. Box 4, Jefferson City, MO 65102
(573) 751-0098   (573) 571-3166 (fax)
www.ecodev.state.mo.us/pr/

Montana Board of Medical Examiners
111 North Jackson Street, Helena, MT 59620-0513
P.O. Box 200513, Helena, MT 59620
(406) 444-4284   (406) 444-1667 (fax)
www.com.state.mt.us/license/pol/main.htm

State of Nebraska Health and Human Services
Registration and Licensure/Credentialing Division
301 Centennial Mall South, Lincoln, NE 68509-4986
P.O. Box 94986, Lincoln, NE 68509-4986
(402) 471-2118   (401) 471-3577 (fax)
www.hhs.state.ne.us/reg/regindex.htm

Nevada State Board of Medical Examiners
1105 Terminal Way, Suite 301, Reno, NV 89502
P.O. Box 7238, Reno, NV 89510
(702) 688-2559   (702) 688-2321 (fax)
www.state.nv.us/medical/

New Hampshire Board of Medicine
2 Industrial Park Drive, Suite 8, Concord, NH 03301-8520
(603) 271-1203   (603) 271-6702 (fax)

New Jersey State Board of Medical Examiners
140 E. Front Street, 2nd Floor, Trenton, NJ 08608
(609) 826-7100, (609) 984-3930 (fax)

New Mexico Board of Medical Examiners
2nd Floor, Lamy Building, 491 Old Santa Fe Trail, Santa Fe, NM 87501
(505) 827-6784   (505) 827-7377 (fax)

New York State Board for Medicine
Cultural Education Center, #3023, Albany, NY 12230
(518) 474-3841   (518) 486-4846 (fax)
www.nysed.gov/prof/profhome.htm

North Carolina Medical Board
1201 Front Street, Suite 100, Raleigh, NC 27609
(919) 828-1212   (919) 326-1131 (fax)
www.docboard.org

North Dakota State Board of Medical Examiners
City Center Plaza, 418 E. Broadway Avenue, Suite 12, Bismarck, ND 58501
(701) 328-6500   (701) 328-6505 (fax)

Ohio State Medical Board
77 S. High Street, 17th Floor, Columbus, OH 43215-6108
(614) 466-3934   (614) 466-4670 (fax)
www.state.oh.us/med/

Oklahoma State Board of Medical Licensure and Supervision
5104 N. Francis, Suite C, Oklahoma City, OK 73118
P.O. Box 18256, Oklahoma City, OK 73154
(405) 848-2189   (405) 848-8240 (fax)
www.osbmls.state.ok.us

Oregon Board of Medical Examiners
1500 S.W. First Avenue, Suite 620, Portland, OR 97201
(503) 229-5770   (503) 229-6543 (fax)
www.bme.state.or.us

Pennsylvania State Board of Medicine
124 Pine Street, Harrisburg, PA 17101
P.O. Box 2649, Harrisburg, PA 17105
(717) 787-2381   (717) 787-7769 (fax)

Rhode Island Department of Health
Board of Medical Licensure and Discipline
Cannon Building, Room 205, 3 Capitol Hill, Providence, RI 02908-5097
(401) 222-3855   (401) 222-2158 (fax)

South Carolina State Board of Medical Examiners
110 Centerview Drive, Suite 202
P.O. Box 11289, Columbia, SC 29211-1289
(803) 896-4500   (803) 896-4515 (fax)
www.llr.sc.edu/me.htm

South Dakota State Board of Medicine And Osteopathic Examiners
1323 S. Minnesota Avenue, Sioux Falls, SD 57105
(605) 336-1965   (605) 336-0270 (fax)

State of Tennessee Department of Health Medical Board
1st Floor Cordell Hull Building
425 5th Avenue North, Nashville, Tn 37247-1010
(615) 532-4384   (615) 532-5369 (fax)
www.state.tn.us/health/

Texas State Board of Medical Examiners
333 Guadeloupe, Tower 3, Suite 610
P.O. Box 2018, Austin, TX 78701
(512) 305-7010   (512) 305-7006 (fax)
www.tsbme.state.tx.us

Utah Division of Ocupational and Professional Licensing
Heber Wells Building, Fourth Floor, 160 E. 300 South
Salt Lake City, UT 84145-0805
(801) 530-6628   (801) 530-6511 (fax)
www.commerce.state.ut.us/

Vermont Board of Medical Practice
109 State Street, Montpelier, VT 05609-1106
(802) 828-2673   (802) 828-5450 (fax)
www.docboard.org

Virginia Board of Medicine
6606 W. Broad Street, 4th Floor, Richmond, VA 23230-1717
(804) 662-9908   (804) 662-9517 (fax)
www.dhp.state.va.us

State of Washington Department of Health
Medical Quality Assurance Commission
P.O. Box 47866, 1300 S.E. Quince Street, Olympia, WA 98504-7866
(360) 236-4785   (360) 586-4573 (fax)
www.doh.wa.gov/hsqa/hpqad/MQAC

West Virginia Board of Medicine
101 Dee Drive, Charleston, WV 25311
(304) 558-2921   (304) 558-2084 (fax)

State of Wisconsin
Department of Regulation and Licensing
1400 E. Washington Avenue, Room 178 P.O. Box 8935
Madison, WI 53703 Madison, WI 53708
(608) 266-2811   (608) 261-7083 (fax)
badger.state.wi.us/agencies/drl/

Wyoming Board of Medicine
211 West 19th Street, Cheyenne, WY 82002
(307) 778-7053   (307) 778-2069 (fax)

*With proper laws in place
doctors will be required to inform women of
Post Tubal Ligation Syndrome.* - sjb

There Should Be a Law

The following is a draft of a proposed legislation.
If you want to see it become a real law, then YOU must take action.
It's easy to do.
Write your State Representative and tell them that you want them to sponsor, co-sponsor, or "vote yes" on an informed consent bill to tubal ligation.
Your letters count!
Use our sample letter below or write your own note.

Dear Representative:

I am a registered voter in your state. I wish to direct your attention to www.tubal.org, the public petition directed to you, and the proposed bill.

I agree that a law is needed to end the practice of doctors withholding information about tubal ligation surgeries.

I ask that you sponsor, co-sponsor, and or endorse a law in our state that would protect women from forced or fraudulent consent to tubal ligation/sterilization.

Sincerely, Jane/John Doe

Draft of Proposed Legislation:

Modernization Act for Women's Informed Consent for Tubal Ligation and Fallopian Tube Devices for Contraception

WHEREAS, tubal ligation and medical devices which affect the fallopian tubes for the purpose of birth control are conceived to be permanent forms of birth control also known as tubal occlusion or sterilization; and,

WHEREAS, all forms of birth control list and disclose both risks and benefits of each expect for sterilization. Information that is withheld from women regarding the side effects of sterilization include information about long term physical and hormonal side effects known commonly as Post Tubal Syndrome (PTS); and,

WHEREAS, Post Tubal Syndrome is known and understood by the medical community but routinely this information is withheld from women. This constitutes forced or fraudulent consent; and,

WHEREAS, some women are nervous while obtaining verbal information from their providers, and or must see and hear information more than once, and or have poor hearing, eyesight, or memories, and or need printed information in hand to discuss with loved ones in order to wage their consent; and

WHEREAS, only with proper laws in place will women be protected from forced or fraudulent consent to sterilization.

BE IT RESOLVED THAT UPON ENACTMENT OF THIS LAW:

It will be the responsibility of the provider performing the sterilization, the hospital/surgical center, and involved insurance companies to ensure the patient is informed in writing.

Providers shall give women "Take-Home-and-Keep Informed Consent" outlining the risks and benefits of tubal ligation upon which to make informed decisions to:

    1. All pregnant women at the time of their first consultation regarding their pregnancy.

    2. All women at the time of their first consultation regarding sterilization.

Hospital/surgical center scheduling departments shall mail "Take-Home-and Keep Informed Consent" at the time the surgery/procedure is scheduled.

Insurance carriers, the day the procedure is pre-certified, shall mail "Take-Home-and Keep Informed Consent" material and the Quality Assurance Review Criteria to the involved insured woman.

Women consenting to medical devices permanently placed on or inside the fallopian tube shall also receive in advance a duplicate of the package insert and full disclosure of the safety studies, FDA approval status, chemical components, device longevity, human body tolerance, manufacturer's/distributor's name, address, phone number, and contact person.

All information shall be in printed form with no need to ask and shall be in the person's native language.

Women signing consent papers for a sterilization procedure or occlusion devise shall be in an unaltered state of consciousness, shall not be in any stage of labor or postpartum euphoria, and shall not be on mind- or emotion-altering drugs.

No one shall provide "consent" for otherwise competent women who ordinarily could give consent themselves but are rendered in an altered, semiconscious, or unconscious state by medication and or are in mental, emotional or physical distress.

No one shall provide surrogate "consent" or involuntary "consent" for a woman without a court order and the woman's knowledge.

The "Take-Home-and-Keep Informed Consent" shall include but not be limited to:

* The type of sterilization to be done or the name of device that will be used.
* The name of the procedure in generally understood words;
* A description of how the procedure will be performed;
* The reason or indications and contraindications for the procedure;
* Whether the procedure is diagnostic, therapeutic, preventative, or cosmetic;
* Expected outcome concerning pain, function, and sensation;
* Possible risks - hormonal, physical, mental, psychological, emotional, and social;
* Possible complications, including infection rates and those documented and provided by the Freedom of Information Act and provided by NLM, PubMed;
* Cost and expense;
* Average recuperation time

The signed legal consent shall name the procedure:
   1. In generally understood words.
   2. By official name, description, and computer code number exactly as it appears in the Current Procedural Terminology book.

The signed legal consent shall name each and every "incidental" procedure, including the creation of disfiguring scars by naming the incision, number, location, and size, i.e., "2-inch horizontal band-aid belly button incision (laparoscopy) which will be closed with invisible stitches under the skin, or visible stitches, visible staples, or skin steri strip tape..."

Consent for "possible" procedures shall state the precise condition requiring the "possible" procedure. The Operative Report shall give clear, cogent, and indisputable photographic documentation of any unforeseen condition/s requiring the consented "possible" procedure/s.

The signed legal consent shall name the primary and all assistant operators by their full legal names and titles; shall clearly identify students/trainees, and whether they are observers or operators; and shall clearly identify procedures new to seasoned practitioners.

The signed legal consent shall state all known/possible benefits and risks including but not limited to:

General information:
  * Sterilization may improve economic status

The risks that can occur with all surgeries in general:
  * General anesthesia risks
  * Risk of infection
  * Risk of adhesions
  * Risk of bleeding
  * Postoperative pain

The risks that can occur specifically with laparoscopic surgery (such as caused by the Veress-needle/Trocar):
  * Intestinal perforation (bowel injuries)
  * Uterine perforation, abdominal wall emphysema, peritonism, mesosalpinx rupture
  * Injury to the major retroperitoneal vessels (injury of a major blood-vessel)

* Perforation of an organ or vessels
* Fallopian tube rupture (tearing of the ovarian tubes)
* Risk of hemorrhages from salpinges on dissected Omentum

The risks relating to the sterilization process (that affecting the fallopian tubes):

* Considered permanent. While reversal is possible in some instances, it is not a guarantee.
* Risk of sterilization failure.
* If sterilization failure occurs then at higher risk of ectopic pregnancy.
* Risk of post-sterilization regret.
* Risk of post tubal syndrome (PTS) (altered ovarian function, menstrual abnormalities)
* Risk of disturbances of menstruation, dyspareunia and altered sexual life.
* Higher risk of subsequent hospital admission for menstrual disorders.
* Increase risk of hysterectomy.
* Risk of ovarian isolation to one or both ovaries (leading to ovarian failure), with explanation why.
* Reduced risk of ovarian cancer, with explanation why.
* Risk of less milk production for lactating women.

Women shall also be informed that:

* The fallopian tube contains hormonal receptor cells, and can not be replaced once removed.
* Sterilization does not protect from AIDS and STDs.

A written test shall document the comprehension of all informed consent material. This will be completed and signed by the woman and will become part of the legal signed consent.

BE IT FINALLY RESOLVED THAT,

Victims of forced, fraudulent, and incomplete informed consent to sterilization will be protected by the full extent of the law.

Victims shall be treated or referred to affordable multidisciplinary physical, mental, emotional, social, financial, legal, and support group help.

It shall be a crime to aid or cover up malfeasance; misrepresent the federal, state, or hospital laws and bylaws; fail to halt, report, acknowledge and validate deviations from standards of care; obstruct justice; refuse to diagnose or treat, dismiss as "normal" or "mentally unstable"; or send victims back to the perpetrator.

A violation of the Legislation shall constitute a reportable misdemeanor. State Medical Boards shall forward all complaints concerning informed consent to sterilization to their State Attorney General. The Attorney General and lawyers shall enforce state law and file suits.

Respectfully submitted by, Susan J Bucher of Lockport, IL

Copyright © 2004 Susan J Bucher and the CPTwomen

ILLINOIS NOW - TUBAL LIGATION RESOLUTION

On 9-25-99, at Illinois NOW's state conference, I presented the following "Tubal Ligation Resolution" - It passed unanimously.

1999 ILLINOIS NOW - TUBAL LIGATION RESOLUTION

WHEREAS, tubal ligation is the number one method of birth control used by women over the age of 30 in the united states; and,

WHEREAS, all forms of birth control list and disclose both risks and benefits of each expect for tubal ligation. Information that is withheld from women regarding the side effects of tubal ligation include information about long term hormonal side effects; and,

WHEREAS, this information is known by the medical community but routinely this information is withheld from women. This constitutes forced or fraudulent consent.

BE IT RESOLVED, that IL NOW support and work with IL Will County NOW in educating the public and other state chapters; and,

BE IT FURTHER RESOLVED, that IL NOW actively recruit and solicit input and activism from post tubal women; and,

THEREFORE BE IT FINALLY RESOLVED, that IL NOW lead the way for other states by lobbying their (IL) state representatives and legislative bodies to put in place proper laws that would protect women when consenting to a tubal ligation.

Respectfully submitted, Susan J Bucher, Will County IL NOW chapter

Information for Researchers:

Books authored by noted physicians who describe post tubal syndrome can be found at: http://home.swbell.net/birons/effects.htm

Noted Articles:

"Post-Tubal Ligation Pain"

From IPPS - Simsbury Connecticut - April/May, 1999

OBGYN.net Editorial Advisors, James Carter, MD and Ahmed El-Minawi, MD, PhD

- Dr. El-Minawi: "...definitely - we believe in post-tubal ligation syndrome. Most of the patients present with menstrual disturbances, usually menorrhagia, menometromenorrhagia, and sorry to say - the majority of the patients ended up as hysterectomy candidates...." "Most of them present anywhere between five to ten years with an average of seven years following the surgery. Most of them have had tubal ligations with destructive tubal ligation types, Pomeroy-type tubal ligations, Irving-type tubal ligations; basically mid-segments tubal ligations are the worst type and are the most causes of post-tubal ligation syndrome."

- Dr. Carter: "...a very high percentage of those women with post-tubal ligation syndrome had adenomyosis." "...this finding of relationship with pelvic congestion after tubal ligation, I believe, is a real problem. So if an individual has had a tubal ligation 5-10 years prior, is experiencing more and more heavy bleeding, is experiencing more and more pain, then in fact, they may have this syndrome."

www.obgyn.net/displaytranscript.asp?page=/avtranscripts/carter_elminawi

Is there such an entity as post tubal ligation syndrome?

After looking at all of the articles both for and against the existence of post tubal ligation syndrome, I have changed my mind. There IS a higher incidence of menstrual dysfunction and noncyclic pain following tubal ligations than the same time progression in women without tubal ligations.

"Premature menopause may be an occasional complication of a sterilization procedure." Frederick R. Jelovsek MD

http://www.wdxcyber.com/nbleed9.htm

Am J Obstet Gynecol. 1992 Jun;166(6 Pt 1):1698-705; discussion 1705-6

Tubal sterilization and risk of subsequent hospital admission for menstrual disorders.

Shy KK, Stergachis A, Grothaus LG, Wagner EH, Hecht J, Anderson G.

Department of Obstetrics and Gynecology, University of Washington, Seattle 98195.

CONCLUSIONS: Tubal sterilization is associated with a greater risk of hospitalization for menstrual disorders.

Am J Epidemiol, 1993 Oct 1, 138:7, 508-21

Long-term risk of hysterectomy among 80,007 sterilized and comparison women at Kaiser Permanente, 1971-1987

Goldhaber MK; Armstrong MA; Golditch IM; Sheehe PR; Petitti DB; Friedman GD

Division of Research, Kaiser Permanente Medical Care Program of Northern California, Oakland 94611.

Findings: Sterilized women were significantly more likely than were comparison women to undergo hysterectomy...

Evaluating the effects of tubal sterilization on menstrual function:

selected issues in data analysis.

Martinez-Schnell B; Wilcox LS; Peterson HB; Jamison PM; Hughes JM

Division of Reproductive Health, Centers for Disease Control, Atlanta, Georgia 30333. Source : Stat Med, 1993 Feb, 12:3-4, 355-63

Marginal modelling resulted in a statistically significant increase in the odds of menstrual dysfunction at 5 years after tubal sterilization.

Obstet Gynecol. 1998 Feb;91(2):241-6.

Higher hysterectomy risk for sterilized than nonsterilized women:

findings from the U.S. Collaborative Review of Sterilization.

The U.S. Collaborative Review of Sterilization Working Group.

Hillis SD, Marchbanks PA, Tylor LR, Peterson HB.

Division of Reproductive Health, National Center for Chronic Disease Prevention and Health Promotion, Centers for Disease Control and Prevention, Atlanta, Georgia 30333, USA.

CONCLUSION: Women undergoing tubal sterilization were more likely than women whose husbands underwent vasectomy to undergo hysterectomy within 5 years after sterilization, regardless of age at sterilization. An increased risk of hysterectomy was observed for each method of tubal occlusion.

J Natl Med Assoc. 2001 Apr;93(4):149-50. PMID: 12653402

Fallopian tube necrosis after postpartum sterilization.

Poma PA, Barber A.

Zentralbl Gynakol. 1989;111(16):1124-7.

The effect of postpartum tubal sterilization on milk production

Vytiska-Binstorfer E.

Universitats-Frauenklinik, Wien.

We investigated 64 women after the so called "post partum sterilization" and recorded also retrospectively the milk production within the first seven days. It was performed by at semilunar subumbilical incision and a bipolar coagulation of the fallopian tubes. The total daily milk production, which was compared with the quantity of milk after the previous pregnancy, was on day six and seven significantly lower after tubal ligation than in the normal puerperal phase before.

J Womens Health Gend Based Med. 2000 Jun;9(5):521-7. PMID: 10883944

Tubal ligation, menstrual changes, and menopausal symptoms.

Visvanathan N, Wyshak G.

Recently, there has been growing evidence that tubal sterilization protects against ovarian cancer, possibly through physiological transformations that result in ovarian dysfunction and decline. This report explores the possibility that the biological mechanism of ovarian dysfunction and decline may affect the menstrual and menopausal changes that result from hormonal imbalances.

http://www.ncbi.nlm.nih.gov/entrez/query.fcgi?cmd=
Retrieve&db=PubMed&list_uids=10883944&dopt=Abstract

Ginecol Obstet Mex. 2002 Jun;70:264-9. Spanish. PMID: 12148467

Relationship of bilateral tubal occlusion with functional ovarian cysts

de Alba Quintanilla F, Posadas Robledo FJ.

"...there is the chance of consequence and long term symptoms and this should be informed to the patient."

http://www.ncbi.nlm.nih.gov/entrez/query.fcgi?cmd=
Retrieve&db=PubMed&list_uids=12148467&dopt=Abstract

Eur J Obstet Gynecol Reprod Biol. 2002 Jan 10;100(2):204-7. PMID: 11750966

The effect of surgical sterilization on ovarian function: a rat model.

Kuscu E, Duran HE, Zeyneloglu HB, Demirhan B, Bagis T, Saygili E.

CONCLUSION: Tubal ligation may affect ovarian function, which in turn may reflect to ovarian histology (menopause) in rats.

http://www.ncbi.nlm.nih.gov/entrez/query.fcgi?cmd=
Retrieve&db=PubMed&list_uids=11750966&dopt=Abstract

Katilolehti. 1998 Jan;103(1):9. Finnish. PMID: 9505666

Late effects of sterilization in women

Sumiala S.

Sterilization exerts a measurable effect on the ovaries,

http://www.ncbi.nlm.nih.gov/entrez/query.fcgi?cmd=
Retrieve&db=PubMed&list_uids=9505666&dopt=Abstract

Obstet Gynecol. 1979 Aug;54(2):189-92.

Luteal deficiency among women with normal menstrual cycles, requesting reversal of tubal sterilization.

Radwanska E, Berger GS, Hammond J.

Reduced midluteal serum progesterone concentration appears more common among women with prior tubal ligation or electrocoagulation than among a control population of apparently normal women.

http://www.ncbi.nlm.nih.gov/entrez/query.fcgi?cmd=
Retrieve&db=PubMed&list_uids=460752&dopt=Abstract

Image J Nurs Sch. 1992 Spring;24(1):15-8.

Post-tubal sterilization syndrome.

Lethbridge DJ.

This article presents a review of the literature on post-tubal sterilization syndrome. Although studies have shortcomings they suggest the majority of women undergoing tubal sterilization do not experience changes in menstrual patterns after the procedure, but a minority do. Suggestions are made for further research, conducted from a nursing perspective. Implications for practice are suggested, given the tentative information on post-tubal sterilization syndrome.

http://www.ncbi.nlm.nih.gov/entrez/query.fcgi?db=PubMed&cmd=Retrieve&list_uids=1541464&dopt=Citation

Adv Contracept. 1994 Mar;10(1):51-6.

Changes in ovarian function after tubal sterilization.

Hakverdi AU, Taner CE, Erden AC, Satici O.

Progesterone levels significantly decreased ($p < 0.001$) and anovulation was observed in 13 (30.2%) of 43 cases. Our data suggest that tubal sterilization carried increased risk in ovarian function, particularly luteal phase deficiency and anovulation.

http://www.ncbi.nlm.nih.gov/entrez/query.fcgi?db=PubMed&cmd=Retrieve&list_uids=8030455&dopt=Citation

TITLE: Risk and contraception: what women are not told about tubal ligation.

AUTHORS: Turney L   SOURCE: WOMEN'S STUDIES INTERNATIONAL FORUM. 1993 Sep-Oct;16(5):471-86.

SECONDARY SOURCE ID: PIP/091715

ABSTRACT: The most common method of fertility control is tubal ligation. Physicians and some women promote tubal sterilization as an extremely safe and very effective method of permanent fertility control. Yet the medical profession has known since 1930 that significant numbers of women suffer serious and irreversible complications from tubal ligations; women have died from tubal ligation. Its mortality rates in Bangladesh, the UK, and US, are 1/5000, 1/10,000, and 1/25,000, respectively. Women experience complications both during and after surgery (e.g., twisting of the tube, sometimes accompanied by gangrene, and accumulation of fluid in a tube). After tubal ligation, many women develop endometriosis.

Torsion, hydrosalpinx, and/or endometriosis contribute to increased menstrual pain. Disturbance of the local flora can cause sepsis (e.g., toxic shock syndrome). Some women have a severe inflammatory reaction to the silicone in clips and rings. Tubal ligation may be linked to an increased risk of cervical cancer. Many sterilized women eventually undergo hysterectomy. Many women experience excessive bleeding during menstruation, but many physicians discount this as women not knowing their own bodies and subjective estimates of blood loss. Impaired ovarian blood supply and altered nerve supply to the tube and/or ovary are possible causes for post-tubal ligation menstruation problems. Many women experience memory loss, general decline in feeling of well-being, lethargy, and loss of libido after tubal ligation, indicating a spontaneous iatrogenic menopause. Yet physicians often attribute these symptoms to psychological problems, thereby denying women knowledge of their own bodies. Tubal ligation-induced problems should not be limited to the medical profession. We need to seriously examine the processes that keep this information from women.

TITLE: Sterilisation of women [letter]

AUTHORS: Dickon S

SOURCE: NEW ZEALAND MEDICAL JOURNAL. 1987 Dec 9;100(837):755.

SECONDARY SOURCE ID: PIP/057531

ABSTRACT: There is some evidence that women who undergo tubal sterilization, especially with cautery techniques, are at greater risk of subsequent hysterectomy. The tubal surgery apparently interferes with the ovary's blood supply, leading to decreased hormonal output, irregular ovulation, and an abnormal pattern of uterine bleeding that becomes the basis for the need for hysterectomy. Given this evidence, it is appalling to find that New Zealand women are being encouraged to undergo tubal ligation without any counseling regarding the chance of heavy bleeding problems within 5-10 years. Moreover, the alternative of having the male partner seek vasectomy is rarely presented. It is the duty of gynecologists to give this problem more attention in pre-sterilization counseling sessions. Useful toward this end would be a leaflet that could be given to patients at the time of their 1st consultation outlining the risks and benefits of tubal ligation.

*Sometimes becoming an activist
and working to make social changes
can help emotional health and healing.
This is the route that I choose
and hope that you can too.* - sjb

In closing - Susan J Bucher 1-29-2006

It is my hope is that one-day a law will be pasted that requires women be informed before TL.

Will I see this in my lifetime?

I have been told no, but have believed that I will.

In seeing how women are treated in other countries, and seeing how our rights are suddenly being striped of us in the US, now I'm not quite sure. I still want to believe that I will.

I'm hoping that women follow through when they say they want to help. I have received thousands of letters. I'm hoping women are also writing to their state reps and media. The actions that are advocated do not cost money, but do take some thought and time.

This book is in no way complete or final. This anthology will be added to and continued… What was not presented in this text is my story and what happened personally to me. My actions have included testifying in person to Senators, writing to State Representatives explaining the need for an informed consent law, suing the doctor who created my condition and the doctor who performed my legendary 2nd surgery (he created false documents to obstruct justice and jeopardize my first legal case), submitting complaints to State medical boards regarding the actions of these doctors, and testifying to State Representatives about the corruption found and ongoing in the State medical boards.

It also doesn't contain information about what happened to Dr. Hufnagel. While many events occurred to her before I met her, I was witness to events and actions that occurred against her since 1997.

There is a strong force of propaganda that there isn't such a beast as post tubal ligation syndrome. There is a force out there trying to create the myth that PTLS is a myth. This force tries to create the dogma that everything that is said and presented here in this book, and everything stated by Dr. Hufnagel is lies. This can be compared to Cassandra and her relationship with Apollo. Explanation will be presented in a future edition, as will be writing exposing the myth makers, which is about the Spin-Doctors, the myths that they have presented and created, and how they "wage the dog".

In order to expand the "Campaign to Inform", Dr. Hufnagel, MD has offered to host national "Healing of Tubal Ligation Syndrome (PTLS)

Workshops" in conjunction with the Health Freedom Expos. She is creating a forum to bring advocates and healers together to speak on the subject of the side effects of tubal ligation surgery, and to work towards physical, emotional, and social healing. These forums allow personal stories to be shared with each other, and helps to educate the public. She is the first doctor ever to offer this type of gathering and educational program in history.

The first meeting and workshop is scheduled to be held Friday 2/24 at 6 PM. For more information about this and upcoming conferences see www.tubal.org or www.DrHufnagel.com. Follow up and meeting minutes will be presented on the web site www.tubal.org as well as the occurrences that take place during these meetings.

Resource web links:

Coalition for Post Tubal Ligation Women - www.tubal.org

Dr. Vikki Hufnagel, MD - www.drhufnagel.com

FSH Test Kits - www.Home-Menopause-Test.com

Health Freedom Expo - www.HealthFreedomExpo.com

To locate your State Representative see:

www.house.gov/house/MemberWWW.shtml

www.house.gov/writerep/

When writing to your representatives, it is advocated that you send a letter rather than e-mail. A tangible letter in the hand can not be deleted or ignored.

Suggested Reading:

Against Their Will
An excellent site explaining North Carolina's Sterilization Program
http://againsttheirwill.journalnow.com/

Claude Moore Health Sciences Library - Eugenics: Three Generations
http://www.healthsystem.virginia.edu/internet/library/historical/eugenics/

Coerced Sterilization of Native American Women
www.geocities.com/CapitolHill/9118/mike.html

Indigenous Women's Reproductive Rights
http://www.nativeshop.org/pro-choice.html

The Straight Dope on the Sterilization of Native Women
http://www.bluecorncomics.com/sterile.htm

Stolen Wombs
Indigenous Women Most at Risk
Bruce E. Johansen
http://www.ratical.org/ratville/stolenWombs.txt

Eugenics movement reaches its height – 1923
Public Broadcasting Service (PBS)
http://www.pbs.org/wgbh/aso/databank/entries/dh23eu.html

War Against The Weak
http://www.waragainsttheweak.com/

The Christian Science Monitor
http://www.csmonitor.com/2006/0118/p25s01-stct.html

Eugenics Watch
http://www.eugenics-watch.com/

Twenty-Five Ways To Suppress Truth: The Rules of Disinformation (Includes The 8 Traits of A Disinformationalist) by H. Michael Sweeney
http://www.whale.to/b/sweeney_h.html

Side Effects of Tubal Ligation Sterilizations
http://home.swbell.net/birons/effects.htm

Iatrogenic Illness: The Downside of Modern Medicine
A White Paper by Gary Null, PhD & Debora Rasio, MD
www.garynull.com/Documents/Iatrogenic/Women/10Hysterectomy.htm